Making Health Teams Work

# Making Health Teams Work

Harold Wise
Richard Beckhard
Irwin Rubin
Aileen L. Kyte

Ballinger Publishing Company • Cambridge, Mass.
*A Subsidiary of J.B. Lippincott Company*

Much of the material in this book was originally prepared as a report to the Carnegie Corporation of New York.



International Standard Book Number: 0–88410–112–6 (cloth)
0–88410–113–4 (paper)

Library of Congress Catalog Card Number: 73–22350

Printed in the United States of America

**Library of Congress Cataloging in Publication Data**

Main entry under title:

Making health teams work.

Bibliography: p.
1. Health services administration. 2. Martin Luther King, Jr. Health Center. I. Wise, Harold. [DNLM: 1. Delivery of health care–U.S. 2. Patient care team. WA525 M235 1974]
RA971.M34 362.1'2 73–22350
ISBN 0–88410–112–6

# Contents

# List of Figures

## List of Tables

# Foreword

As our society begins to show signs of moving, however slowly, from a competitive to a cooperative model, ideas that have lain dormant because they were not congruent with accepted philosophy and practice are beginning to come to the surface. One such idea is a team operation used in the delivery of medical care services.

So long as medical care was the unique province of the single professional in solo practice, dealing directly with his patient, the concept of team practice was anathema, even though the steady multiplication of specialties, the splitting off of one after another professional group from the central physician role, has made the need for teamwork obvious for almost a century. Indeed, cooperative arrangements have long been necessary for the patient's welfare, and provide the appropriate method for effective care of the sick. No matter; the idea was unwelcome. And while sporadic efforts at creating team structures in hierarchic and autocratic design were modestly successful, medical education and tradition continued to foster independent practice. Even when hospital teamwork was lauded, it was permitted only so long as the physician retained control, gave direction, and made the final decision; with this proviso, the cluster of ancillary workers was acceptable.

Despite the constraints, a variety of sources have fostered some small current of counteraction. First, the attenuation of physicians in the public health field enlarged the role and the importance of public health nursing. Second, the unwillingness of physicians to make home calls further strengthened the role of the public health nurse and the role of the social worker, who was often used in conjunction with physicians' services in outpatient care in hospitals. Third, the effect of salaried physicians was to reduce their attachment to many things that they would otherwise have considered essential elements of their role. Everett Hughes, in his book *Men and Their Work,* points out that as responsibilities multiply in a professional movement a kind of subtle and unspoken cost-benefit analysis takes place. The professional tends to shed portions of his job, thereby strengthening the role of the next in line in the hierarchy of service. However, in all these situations the essential hierarchic element remains. The physician is still in charge.

In the late 1950s, in the Family Health Maintenance Demonstration at Montefiore, we were early pioneers in the use of interdisciplinary teams to provide comprehensive patient care. In an effort to overcome the problems of physician dominance, we tried to create a Quaker "sense of the meeting" approach to decision making. The effort only partly succeeded because it failed to deal with the necessity of unifying and strengthening the training of the natural colleagues of the physicians in the health delivery system, which might have created the professional pride necessary to put these health professionals on an equal footing with the physician.

Yet we must recognize there are certain dangers in liberating subordinates and providing them an identity as equals. Professional groups—nurses and social workers as well as physicians—have a tendency to become chauvinistic. Whereas at one time the problem was to create a basis for interaction in which the positive elements of the training and experience of each professional could be maximized for the patient's benefit by allowing each profession in the health delivery system to have a responsible and prideful role, the problem today, as I see it, is to prevent overtraining, overcertification, and magnification of individual roles. When Sir Theodore Fox talked of the "greater medical profession" and of replacing the "kingdom" of medicine with a commonwealth, did he visualize the recrudescence of nationalism as well? It is to be hoped that the concept of team training will help to overcome this parochial development and create a democratic collegial atmosphere. Both patients and professionals must benefit then.

The purpose of this book is to help institutions in the health care field recognize and accept the values implicit in health team operation and to assist them in coping with the problems that they will face in the creation of tomorrow's health service. The team is an indispensable way of delivering modern health services. The training of the team is an indispensable way of assuring that that kind of service works.

**George A. Silver**
*Professor of Public Health*
Yale University, School of Medicine
November 1973

# Preface

The making of a book, even a small one, requires inputs from many people. This book is no exception. To begin at the beginning, the story of the Dr. Martin Luther King, Jr. Health Center obviously could not have been written if the center did not exist. And without funding from the federal government's Office of Economic Opportunity and the support of Dr. Martin Cherkasky, Director of Montefiore Hospital and Medical Center, it would not exist today. Nor would the organization development inputs provided by the consultants from the Sloan School of Management have been possible without benefit of a Carnegie Foundation grant. Generous thanks go to all those who have supported the center.

Basically, the Martin Luther King, Jr. Health Center, like any organization, is its people. For me at least, coming from the business world where the people side of organization often gets preempted by such concepts as return on investment, earnings per share, cost-benefit analysis, asset management, and so on, the center truly provided a breath of fresh air. The willingness of MLK employees, from top management down to the newest trainee, to share their experiences, their feelings, their hopes, fears, and dreams was also essential to the making of this book.

Nor could it have come into being without Harold Wise's determination. For me, working with him has been a challenge. His need for results (preferably instant ones) met head-on my need, barely articulated in the early stages of the project, for something more than just another collection of loosely conjoined articles. The resulting dialectic was, I suspect, important in shaping this project. I want to thank Harold for permitting the necessary gestation period, especially since it must often have seemed as though the birth had been unduly delayed.

I also want to say a special word of thanks to Mrs. Estelle Wallack, formerly Harold Wise's secretary. Many competent people, over the years, have translated my impossibly-marked-up copy into clean manuscript. But no one has ever done this job with Estelle's capability. Her almost intuitive sense of what all the squiggles, arrows, insertions, deletions meant was invaluable in producing this book.

A special word of thanks goes also to Carl Fagin, who shepherded this project through its critical later stages.

Finally, it has been my privilege, as editor of *Making Health Teams Work,* to have been involved in the project from its inception. I thank all those who made this possible, especially Dick Beckhard, from whom I first heard about the Martin Luther King Center and its ongoing work with organization development.

**Aileen L. Kyte**

# Introduction

This book is a record of the efforts of many people to develop a team approach to family-centered health care at the Dr. Martin Luther King, Jr. Health Center (known familiarly as MLK) located in the Morrisania section of the South Bronx, an area where the morbidity and mortality rates of the largely Black and Puerto Rican population are among the highest in New York City. While this is the story of MLK—and as such describes the problems, successes and failures of one health center—the lessons to be learned, we believe, are applicable to any health organization which is attempting to mobilize the efforts of various specialists into a team activity organized around the needs of patients and their families.

Simply put, the theme of our book is the conjunction of the team approach to family health care and the organization development concepts as put forth by a group of consultants headed by Richard Beckhard from the Sloan School of Management of the Massachusetts Institute of Technology. The book is organized into five chapters. Although each is authored independently, the book has a story line—a beginning, a middle, and, we believe, a future rather than an ending.

In Chapter One, in effect, I set the scene for what is to come. Within the context of MLK's early years, I have described how the teams evolved from a disease oriented medical model consisting of physicians and their assistants to a client-centered model that makes use of an interdisciplinary team with medical, nursing, psychological, dental, social, legal, educational, and community development skills all being called on in the struggle to provide comprehensive care on the basis of need as defined by the families being served.

In writing this history of MLK's early years, I have attempted to give the reader a sense of our continuing efforts to define the nature of the basic problem that was preventing us from achieving our goal of a new kind of patient care; of our many attempts, often abortive, to improve the primary care team's functioning; and finally of our finding in the field or organization development a concept as well as a method that we could use to help the teams help themselves to work more effectively.

In essence we became aware of the simple yet powerful notion that a health team needs training to help it work as a team. Irv Rubin, one of the MIT consultants who worked with us, put it so well:

> It is naïve to bring together a highly diverse group of people and expect that, by calling them a team, they will in fact behave as a team. It is ironic indeed to realize that a football team spends 40 hours a week practicing teamwork for the two hours on Sunday afternoon when their teamwork really counts. Teams in organizations seldom spend two hours per year practicing when their ability to function as a team counts 40 hours per week.

In Chapter Two, the reader can view organization development at work in two of the eight primary care health teams. The process of helping the teams move toward more open communication, a better definition of the roles of various health workers on the teams, and the need to deal with conflict more directly are three of the issues involved in the first MIT intervention. Authors Rubin, Fry, and Lech describe the tasks that the health teams worked on to help them better understand their own dynamics as well as the action-research model the consultants used in planning and carrying out this pilot intervention.

The impact of this work, which involved six of the eight health teams before it was concluded, had repercussions throughout the organization. Most important, it forced MLK's top management to recognize that the center's traditional authoritarian structure had to be changed if the administrative system was to adequately support the teams carrying out their primary care functions. Decisions made at the top of the organization—particularly when we lacked adequate information concerning what went on at other levels—were simply not responsive to the needs of the health teams.

The design of an organization structure that would adequately support the work of the teams is the subject of Chapter Three. Here, Richard Beckhard describes what the team method of health care requires from the overall administrative structure. Within this context, he looks at roles, decision making, power distribution, and staff education. The issues he raises, I believe, have implications for those who provide health services in hospitals and ambulatory centers as well as for those concerned with the education of health workers.

Just as in the case of a single health examination, a single intervention, no matter how successful, will not maintain an organization's health. What must be developed is a self-renewing capability, an internal resource in organization development. In Chapter Four, Aileen Kyte describes the building of such a capability at the MLK Health Center. Part of the chapter is a picture of the OD training program as seen from her perspective as a member of the training group. The anxieties, frustrations, and finally the insights she experienced are typical of experiential training; they occur in work oriented groups, which this group was, as well as in groups primarily concerned with personal growth. It is important, we believe, that managements recognize the kinds of time and energy inputs that such a program requires if it is to be successful in training potential change agents who will help the organization move toward its goal of becoming self-renewing.

Chapter Five looks to the future of health team development. It comprises two papers that describe on-going work. The paper on the Institute for Health Team Development at Montefiore examines the educational strategies and curricula that will be tested on interdisciplinary teams of health science students and faculty. The work of the MIT group is outlined in the second paper, including the testing of team intervention materials which can be self-administered, with minimum use of outside consultation.

Finally, it is our hope that this book will point a direction for health team members, wherever they may be, in their attempts to learn to work together interdependently with the patients and families they serve. If we have charted a direction, we will have succeeded in our goal. All we can add is, "Welcome aboard!"

**Harold Wise**

## About Chapter One

*The year is 1966. The Great Society is moving into high gear. Enthusiasm in Washington is contagious; poverty will be eliminated; discrimination is on the way out. With Job Corps and Head Start already launched, the OEO is now exploring the feasibility of demonstrating high-quality health care in poor communities. "In" phrases are preventive medicine, family-centered care, community involvement, and health teams.*

*Against this backdrop, what was later to become the Dr. Martin Luther King, Jr. Health Center came into being, born of great need, great expectations and great disenchantment with the traditional forms of medical care being offered in poor communities.*

*Dr. Harold Wise, founder and first director of the MLK Center, takes us back to the early struggles to assemble staff, to find a suitable location, and to provide top quality, comprehensive, family-centered care to the inhabitants of Health Districts 24 and 26 in the South Bronx. The vehicle for delivering primary care was to be an interdisciplinary health team, made up of community people as well as doctors and nurses.*

*On paper it seemed reasonable enough; in reality the problems were staggering. On a particularly bad day when a visitor asked Dr. Wise about the optimum size of a team, he replied, "The smaller the better. One is perfect." Obviously, a way had to be found to help the teams work more effectively if the center's faith in the team delivery of health care was to be vindicated.*

*Chapter One, in essence, chronicles this search for help. Did the answer lie in a new breed of social medicine physician? A different kind of nurse practitioner? A community-based family health worker? Or was there some factor that transcended the individual health workers, that had to do with the whole becoming more than the sum of its parts. In Chapter One, we see the concept of teamness and the experience of a team as an entity beginning to emerge.*

## Chapter One

# Evolution of the Health Team: The First Five Years

*Harold Wise*

As I look back over the first five years of the Dr. Martin Luther King, Jr. Health Center project I am impressed with the many milestones that have marked our progress, despite the enormous hurdles we had to overcome. What in concept began as a hospital-based group practice, in five years evolved into a complex health care delivery system, a training center, and a community development project.

In this chapter I want to focus on the evolution of the health team as a means of providing family-centered, comprehensive, sensitive health care in a poor community. To better understand how the team concept developed at MLK, I will try to link my perceptions of the teams' evolution while tracing the history of the project.

This is a personal record, based on my own experience as director of the center. It is also an incomplete record—both in the sense that it is personal and because I make no attempt here to cover every aspect of the program. To do that would be a book in itself.

During the years at MLK I kept a journal, from which I will quote from time to time. My hope is that this will give the reader a more graphic sense of what was involved in our attempt to build a team-oriented health care delivery system and of the overwhelming odds against succeeding that we faced on what seemed to be almost a daily basis.

## INCUBATION

The Neighborhood Medical Care Demonstration (as the Dr. Martin Luther King, Jr. Health Center project was originally called) grew out of the increasingly serious problems Montefiore Hospital in the North Bronx had in providing ambulatory care services at Morrisania City Hospital when the two became affiliated in 1961. Morrisania at that time serviced an impoverished section of the South

Bronx with a high percentage of Black and Puerto Rican families whose morbidity and mortality rates were and are among the highest in New York City. Large numbers of these people were using the emergency room and clinics of Morrisania for their only medical care, overburdening both the facilities and the staff.

Dr. George A. Silver, who was then chief of social medicine at Montefiore, learned of these conditions after the affiliation. In an attempt to relieve the overcrowding as well as to provide more adequate and efficient medical care to the most frequent users of the emergency room and clinics, he developed a plan for a hospital-based group practice at Morrisania in the early 1960s. However, he was not able to get the necessary financing for such an operation.

Late in 1965 I became director of ambulatory services at Morrisania, with responsibility for the home care program, the 60 specialty clinics, and the emergency room. As George Silver had recognized, the situation was grim. The ER, instead of having to care for 50 severely ill persons (for which it was designed), now was attempting to serve 400 persons a day—many of them with minor complaints that usually are handled in a physician's office. The house staff doctors resented not only the patient overload but what they considered an inappropriate use of the emergency room. For me, the dingy, depressing surroundings and the 30-year-old sign appearing in English and Yiddish, warning that employees accepting bribes are subject to firing, bespoke of facilities that had long since become wholly inadequate and of a system that was no longer viable. Not even my first contact with patients on the wards in medical school was as upsetting as the scene at Morrisania.[1]

The 60 specialty clinics were perhaps even worse than the ER. While they had not experienced the phenomenal growth in patient population of the ER (patients avoided them when possible), they were not meeting patient needs. In the early years it was assumed all patients would have a personal physician who would give them the bulk of their medical care, with the clinic used only for consultation or treatment which required hospital services. Now, of course, patients had no personal physician and often sought treatment for multiple problems rather than a single ailment. An elderly man, for example, who had heart disease, diabetes, and arthritis, would have to appear at the cardiac clinic on Monday, the arthritis clinic on Tuesday, and the diabetes clinic on Friday, with each of these visits taking approximately four hours. Even worse than the long waits and fragmented care that patients received was the fact that no one was responsible for coordinating such care. A patient's heart might be treated, his lungs might be treated, his arthritic hands might be treated, but he, an entity, a human being, was never treated.

With a freeze on all further spending, I asked myself what could be done without money? At the very least, it seemed, some of the clinics could be reorganized to treat the patient whatever his ailments. After discussing this with clinic staffs, after several weeks of preparation, after a final memo alerting staff to the date for the changeover, half the clinics were to deal with any and all problems the patient presented.

What happened?

Basically nothing changed. When I confronted the physicians with failure to comply, they smiled, apologized, said they did not understand. But it was clear that what I was up against was something quite different from misunderstanding; something connected, I believe, with the training a physician undergoes. Since inappropriate training for family-centered ambulatory care has played a critical role in the evolution of the MLK health teams, as well as in creating the new internship and residency program in social medicine and the new Institute for Health Team Development, I want to look at physician training briefly in terms of my own experience.

## PHYSICIAN TRAINING—A PIECE AT A TIME

Most medical school students are first placed on anatomy. Practically the only social contact I had for my first year was a cadaver. The second year, pathology—the study of diseased organs of the cadaver. Later in that year we learned parts of the process of physical examination. With black wax pencil we outlined patients' lungs, after carefully percussing them out. Ten of us would line up to listen to one good heart murmur. A piece at a time. A lung, the fundus of an eye, a heart, an abdomen. During the third and fourth years we began to bring these pieces together and some of us, at the end of the fourth year, would do a complete history and physical.

We were taught by specialists. Very few of us tried to deal with the patient as a person or even with all his problems. Often we were encouraged to focus on just one problem for concentrated learning, referring other problems to other specialty clinics. The social aspects of medical care were either taught in public health or psychiatry. We had great contempt for public health, showing up only to prepare for exams. Our focus was on disease, the rarer the better.

When we arrived in the emergency room, as interns, we were disease oriented. Here we were to pick up the technique of dealing with the severely ill. For example, the response was vigorous to a patient with cardiac arrest. An alarm in the hospital would be sounded and a horde of doctors, horn-rimmed, would descend on the patient, thumping on chest, respiring, pouring magic fluids into veins, monitoring the whole process with a snake-like winding of EKG paper, blood samples drawn from various areas, an electric shock given periodically—with relish. But deal with a minor problem, an emotional problem? There was no professional satisfaction. A social worker could do that.

Looking at it this way, no wonder many of the house staff felt that patients were "abusing" the emergency room, using it like a doctor's office, since they were not *really* sick. No wonder, too, the reorganization of the clinics never got off the ground.

Feeling frustrated and angry, I immersed myself in the day-to-day problems of running Morrisania's ambulatory services—filling in for missing doctors, dealing with acute emergencies, signing hundred of requests, making up schedules, getting transportation for patients who could not get home, handling unending complaints. Everything in the situation seemed to work against an effective operation; everything seemed to work against good patient care.

## OEO IN THE PICTURE

During this time I continued my contact with George Silver, who had accepted a position as deputy secretary of the Department of Health, Education, and Welfare. The Johnson years were in full swing now. Legislation was being ground out. Under Sargent Shriver's direction, the Office of Economic Opportunity was gaining momentum. Although the situation was chaotic, enthusiasm was high. Few people doubted that poverty would be eliminated; the questions were merely which way and how long would it take.

Head Start and the Job Corps had already been launched. Now OEO was beginning to explore the possibility of demonstrating comprehensive health services in poor communities. The agency was looking for innovative methods that stressed prevention, family-centered care, and community involvement. Soon after this, Tufts Medical School received a sizable grant to set up a health center at Columbia Point, an isolated low income housing project in Boston.

Perhaps George Silver's proposal for a Morrisania group practice now had a chance. Perhaps if we included some of the new rhetoric calling for "maximum feasible community participation" and "training programs for community people," we could get funding. Under George Silver's careful guidance, I began to rewrite the proposal.

In March 1966, with the proposal rewritten, I paid a visit to Washington. Ms. Lee Bamberger (Schorr), acting director of the health office, greeted me. To George Silver and me the proposal was a way to revolutionize the delivery of medical care. Lee Bamberger's commitment suggested something more. Health was to be the entering wedge; a health center could be the focus for the social rehabilitation of a whole neighborhood. If a community was organized around health issues, why not around housing, around education? It was a way to break the vicious cycle of poverty. While this may seem an almost naïve belief today, at the time it appeared to be a realizable goal and one I found enormously exciting.

OEO liked our proposal; now they wanted a detailed, realistic budget. I went to work with Abe Miller, the Montefiore comptroller who is a genius at translating fantasies into operational realities. On our next visit to OEO, we brought bagels—from the only bagel factory remaining in the Bronx! They were delighted. We were delighted. Guidelines could be changed; red tape was to be eliminated.

The four components of the program were spelled out more clearly:

1. To provide comprehensive health services to families using a team of doctors, nurses, and social workers.
2. To train neighborhood people as health workers in the center.
3. To mobilize community interest around health issues, develop health clubs on each block, and a neighborhood advisory board to provide the "maximum feasible participation" component.
4. To evaluate the program and its costs, to see if it could be demonstrated on a larger scale.

We had requested $2.2 million. In July the word came through that we would get $1.9 million. In August we were funded. After "thinking poor" for so long at Morrisania, the prospect of having sufficient money to set up our project was heady indeed.

Looking back at the proposal and trying to recapture my own state of mind at the time, it seems fairly clear that the idea that community people might have as much to teach the professionals as vice versa had not occurred to me. What was true then and remains true today are the feelings of myself and some of my colleagues expressed in the lead paragraphs of that proposal:

> The poor in America have had little share in the benefits of modern medicine; characteristically their medical care has been fragmented, episodic, and anachronistic. Should they survive their births, they are drawn into a pernicious cycle. It starts with slum living, with inadequate diet and health maintenance; it leads to illness prolonged by lack of medical care and environmental deprivation; it results in loss of income and jobs, thereby forcing the poor into ever more blight. Next to heart disease and cancer, poverty is described as '. . . the third leading cause of death.'[2]
>
> At the present time, the costly, inadequately structured outpatient departments engender feelings of apathy and futility in the community and attitudes of defeatism among the servicing professionals. Tentative approaches toward solution of the problem of the medical-care needs of low income families have tended to be a cautious tinkering with the status quo. It is time that a more imaginative approach toward consolidation of community agency efforts and provision of a more modern systematic organization of service is attempted.
>
> The demonstration-research project aims to attack the health problems of the poor in such a manner. This means providing the

best available medical care—comprehensive, hospital-affiliated group practice that is family-centered; recruiting local doctors and nonmedical personnel who can communicate with the neighborhood inhabitants. It involves organizing the community to stimulate interest and to mobilize the neighborhood in improving its medical care. It confronts the self-perpetuating problem of the unemployed by creating a training program that leads to employing neighborhood nonprofessionals in the provision of health services.

At the time we stated these lofty objectives we had no real idea of how incredibly difficult our attempts to implement them would be.

## EARLY ENTHUSIASM AND RAPID ACHIEVEMENT

The first year of operation was one of enormous excitement, intense anxiety, and significant achievement. Within two months I had assembled most of the key core staff,[3] all of whom were vigorous proponents of their own disciplines and stars in their own right. The goals of the program were sufficiently broad to permit each member of the core staff to see them in terms of his or her own interests and needs. My own goal, of course, was to get the health care part of the program in operation as quickly as possible, with training, community development, and research rating secondary priorities. But all the staff felt pressured by OEO to get into operation, particularly since the Tufts program had set an impossible standard by becoming operational in four to five months.

In August, the same month in which we received the grant, Ron Brooke, our research director, began a door-to-door survey which eventually was to reach every household in the area, including an enormous low income housing project and some of the poorest tenements in New York City. He was as much interested in community development and in the positive effects face-to-face communication would have in community organization as he was in the research results of the activity. In effect this set the stage for a continuing conflict among members of our small group around the philosophy of community organization, which in turn set a pattern for the relationships within the group. For a time, however, our excitement and commitment to the overall project overrode personal rivalries.

That August we also began holding small meetings with community people in neighborhood apartments to explain our program and answer questions. This was my first confrontation with the difficulties of communicating with neighborhood people, who, I soon learned, came from a different world. When I talked about group practice and family medical care, they looked puzzled or skeptical. When I talked about prevention, they asked if the clinic would be open all night. (Not "clinic," we said, "health center.") When members of the core group talked about nonprofessionals involved in the provision of care, community people worried whether nonprofessionals would be used to replace doctors. We were surprised at their priorities. Jobs (money) was first. Then housing—could we help improve enforcement of the housing code? Then police protection—did the hospital have any influence with the Mayor? With all the stories of police brutality, we were surprised they wanted cops on every block (on foot, not in the cars). And then came transportation. Would we do house calls? Would we provide transportation to and from the health center?

Education and preventive medical care were low priorities—except for dental care. Only a small percentage of the most severely affected children had received any dental care. And no one will hire you with bad teeth, they told us. Clearly we had a lot to learn and a lot of educating to do if our health care concepts were to mean anything in the community.

During these early months we operated out of one crowded, noisy room in Morrisania. We were bitterly disappointed in October when the city refused to approve the necessary renovations needed to set up temporary medical care facilities at the hospital, which set back the medical part of the program many months.

That winter, after much searching, we finally located what seemed to be the only suitable building in the area for housing our project—an old five-story warehouse on Third Avenue under the El, which Montefiore then purchased. Originally we anticipated moving into our new quarters the following November. However, since two floors were occupied, closure was delayed for many months. When it became clear that the main center could not be ready until some time in 1968, we leased a burned-out five and dime store ("Cheap Charlie's") on Bathgate Avenue. After extensive renovation, it would operate as a neighborhood health center and eventually as a satellite to our main center. But renovation here was also delayed, this time by a local plumbers' strike.

Despite these frustrations, we were busy planning our two new facilities and dealing with the myriad problems connected with the powerful bureaucracies—city, state, federal, and Montefiore—through which we had to operate.

## FOCUS ON TRAINING

While the medical part of the program was running into a series of roadblocks, research, training, and community development were moving ahead. Stella Zahn, our training director, was the first to break loose. She had located some space in the huge housing project in the district we were to serve and announced one morning that in three weeks she planned to start the training program. Everyone was stunned. "We don't have the health center yet—how can we start training?" I asked. But Stella was firm. If our center couldn't hire her "graduates," she would find other sites for them.

She had definite ideas of what she was about. She felt that on-the-job training programs had failed in the past because people opted for a job before they were ready for work and before they were aware of what the job entailed; hence the 50–75 percent dropout rate. She also felt that training had been directed primarily to the young, who had not yet settled down. By bringing in an older group, training would take on a more serious tone.

We were all shocked when Stella insisted that a time clock be installed—that trainees had to punch in and punch out. If people were to learn to hold down a job, she said, they would have to conform. And call in when sick. And if they were late three times, it meant out. (We were very ambivalent about strictness, for inevitably it meant that the most needy dropped out.)

We had decided that all trainees must live in the geographic area we would serve, with preference given to those on welfare and heads of households. Each trainee was to be paid a stipend of $55 a week during training.

When the word got out in the community, more than 150 people applied for the 30 training slots. Selection was difficult and painful. We finally ended up with 26 people who seemed like good risks and four (two ex-addicts and two women on welfare with large numbers of children) who looked shaky. From the beginning we were ambivalent about taking the best (who would probably succeed without us) versus taking the neediest. But it became clear early on that one needs more than a modicum of the middle class ethos to function in a health facility. So we soon dropped the idea of trying to train the severely hard core—delaying that issue. I wrote at the time:

> Preparations for the first day are frantic, with all of us involved. The textbooks were ordered too late. There is no toilet paper. How are we to get everybody into two rooms!
>
> The trainees arrive. There are the opening speeches. We love them. They love us. We are going to turn the training business upside down. We are on our way.
>
> Actually the first eight weeks are trial and probe. The trainees are anxious to get into on-the-job training, yet Stella sticks to the pre-job core. By the fourth week half the class has changed their minds about the kinds of jobs they want, when they get some insights into the actual work content. At the end of the eighth week, 26 of the 30 graduate. (Using our present criteria, we would have dropped three others.) Stella does a great job of placing most of them in on-the-job training spots.

It was clear to us now that training was going to be one of our most important activities for it meant a job, money—the highest priority of community people. But it also meant anger, disappointment, hostility—since for every applicant accepted, ten were turned down. Inevitably we were accused of favoritism in our selection process. And although we later included local resident on the selection committee, the center's training program continued as a valuable yet controversial activity.

## THE EMERGENCE OF TEAMS

During this whole time I was rethinking my own experience with the home care team at Montefiore and what George Silver had told me about his experience with the family health maintenance demonstration project, which also made use of health teams. I reread his book, *Family Medical Care,*[4] and, feeling it had special significance for our project; circulated copies to all top team members. Since both these projects were to play an important role in the evolution of health teams at MLK, I will briefly describe them.

The home care team, set up in the late 1940s by Dr. Martin Cherkasky, was devised as a way to provide medical services in the home to patients whose problems had already been investigated and stabilized in the hospital but who no longer required hospital care. The patients, most of whom were elderly and chronically ill, had to have family or other homemaking support to qualify for home care assistance. The home care team consisted of an internist, who saw the patient once or twice a month; a public health nurse, who visited the home more often; and a social worker, who handled any problems connected with social agencies.

Although the physician was supposedly in charge of the teams, the nurse really ran the show. Patients would contact her directly and she handled a lot of day-to-day problems as well as nursing duties. The team, which uses the hospital model except for the nurse's expanded role, is considered an effective one.

This was my first experience with a health team.

George Silver's family health maintenance demonstration at Montefiore had much broader goals (some of which were similar to those we had set for the health center): preventive and curative services were offered—in the home, ambulatory unit, and hospital—to 150 middle income families to promote their physical and emotional well-being. In the demonstration, the basic team was made up of an internist, a pediatrician, a public health nurse, a social worker and a secretary; a psychiatrist, psychologist, and health educator were available when needed.

In the course of discussing George Silver's health maintenance demonstration project with the core group, our own delivery system began to take form. The team that we envisioned initially was to be made up of a general practitioner who would act as a family doctor, a public health nurse and a social worker. We did not see community people as part of the health team at that point, although they would be trained to do a variety of tasks to assist the professionals.

But several factors were to force us to modify this structure. To begin with, while the salaries we offered were the same as in the hospital, I could find few general practitioners who were interested in working in an ambulatory care center in a run-down, low income area. For this reason, as well as my own bias, I quickly moved to the split I had been trained in, of internists and pediatricians.

Also my ambivalence toward social workers came to the fore—reinforced by Dr. Silver's experience in the family health maintenance demonstration. In his teams, the social worker had been the least acceptable member. So while I went through the motions of interviewing a few social workers, I was starting to think in another direction. I had recently read a theoretical article on a multipurpose health worker. Instead of a social worker, I thought, why not train a community person to do many health related tasks. Such a health worker, who understood family problems, might serve as a needed link on the health teams between our professional staff and the people in the community.

## ENTER THE FAMILY HEALTH WORKER

The top group responded enthusiastically to the concept of a family health worker, each person tending to see this new paraprofessional as an extension of his or her capabilities. Harriet Bograd, the lawyer in the group, said the family health worker ought to be a kind of community lawyer and she wrote a strong position paper stating that this new health worker should be trained in advocacy skills. Another member said the family health worker should be taught to be useful around the home, to fix broken plumbing, repair defective wiring, that kind of thing. This also became part of the job—at least on paper. The nursing component was more traditionally conceived: the family health worker was to be trained pretty much as a practical nurse or nurse's aide. Health education and community development were also to be her responsibilities, as we envisioned her role. Thinking back, it was a little like an elephant being put together by people who are specialists in the tail, the trunk, the legs, etc.

Beyond the fact of requiring multiple and often dissimilar capabilities, the trouble (which we didn't recognize until later) was that the medical personnel—the doctors and the nurses who would be supervising and working with this new paraprofessional—had no input into or say about what training she should have or what her job should be. So right from the beginning the family health worker role emerged as the center of conflict. At the time, however, we felt the family health worker alone would be the answer to many of the insensitivities encountered in the traditional rendering of medical care.

The job of developing a curriculum for the family health worker's on-the-job training was delegated to a nurse in the medical department who, it turned out, was basically opposed to the important role we had planned for this paraprofessional. At the time, however, because of my concern with getting the center on stream, I failed to recognize the impact of her attitude. She was a competent nurse, intelligent, well liked by the staff. Surely it would work out.

It didn't. When the eight community people who had already gone through the eight-week core program (which stressed basic health skills, community resources, and remedial courses in English and mathematics), reported to work, there was no curriculum. We had seven vociferous women and one man who didn't know what they were going to be trained to do by a group of doctors and nurses who didn't know how to train them, and who, in some cases, were opposed to their role altogether.

What to do?

After a series of discussions with the nurse I concluded that the program would never work under her jurisdiction. So I asked Fuller Torrey, one of the physicians working closely with me, to take on the training assignment. Then, after some terrible soul searching, I asked the nurse to resign. Firing anyone has always been extraordinarily painful for me. It means that I literally and figuratively take away that person's bread; and in retribution I lose a bit of my gut. Those who say that you are doing the person a favor when you fire him, etc., etc. have provided little solace—I simply don't believe them.

In this instance, besides my personal feelings, repercussions were immediate and serious, both among the staff and in the neighborhood. People stopped talking when I entered a room. I was called a racist. I faced a large sit-down strike by the staff and a picketing by some angry neighborhood residents. For a while it looked as though the whole project might go under. And although we managed to hold on, the scars of this episode remained visible for many months. I myself was deeply depressed by what had happened.

## NEW ROLES FOR NURSES

The family health worker's training was not the only training problem we faced that winter as we pushed ahead toward the opening of Bathgate in June. The nurse's role on the team was also far from clear. While no one felt she should be limited to a traditional nursing role, we had not thought through what her expanded responsibilities should be. Around Christmas our research director had come back from visiting Dr. Henry Silver's program in Denver where they were successfully training nurses as practitioners. We sent two of our nurses out there to get their reactions and they were genuinely excited. All right, we said, we'll train nurses as primary care practitioners. And then, possibly because of the nurse's role in the home care teams and the fact that they had successfully coordinated the work on George Silver's health maintenance teams, as a needed boost to their morale I suggested they should be the team leaders.

So within a very brief time the role of the team nurse moved from a traditional perspective to having responsibility for three key areas: the nurses were to supervise the newly trained family health workers; they were to be trained as nurse practitioners; and they were assigned the team leadership role.

Our new breed of nurse, like our family health workers, we felt, would be an important part of the answer to providing the kind of sensitive family-centered care we had planned.

## BATHGATE OPENS

As we approached the opening of Bathgate in early June we were euphoric. "Cheap Charlie's" had been transformed into a small modern health center, with good equipment, comfortable furniture, a lab, an X-ray unit, and a tiny pharmacy. Compared to the other clinics around, the place was a honey. Colorful, bright, and cozy, it was tangible proof of our success.

But when the patients started arriving, my anxiety became acute. I ran around frantically, becoming extremely critical of staff if a patient had even a five minute wait. Dr. William B. Lloyd, the medical director and my friend, took me firmly by the arm; he said things would take a few days to settle down, and in the meantime I'd better disappear. I felt an enormous burden lift.

Almost from the beginning we organized ourselves into teams. The primary health team consisted of two nurses, an internist, a pediatrician, and four to six family health workers. A social scientist and a lawyer were available to the teams on a consulting basis. The teams worked the same sessions and held a team conference once a week. Although the nurses had been delegated the role of team leader, the doctors actually ran things. But no one seemed to mind. Our shared sandwich lunches seemed to express the egalitarian feelings of the group.

Looking back, I realize it was Bill Lloyd who had a far clearer concept of team operation than I did at the time. He seemed to know instinctively what to do to make a team work. He was also indispensable in organizing our record keeping and setting up the appointment system.

We had recognized that facilities at Bathgate could not accommodate all the people in the area which we eventually hoped to serve. In consultation with our community advisory board, we had developed a plan for limited registration. By the end of the first week we were seeing 60 patients a day (our early projected limit). By the end of the first month we were seeing 100 a day.

Our goal was to have every family assigned to a health team. The teams, with the family's active cooperation, would develop a comprehensive health plan for each family. Appointments, as needed, would be made with the appropriate team member. Medical records of all family members would be kept together in a binder. The family would know whom to contact and where to come when any member needed help. In this way we could truly provide comprehensive, continuing family-centered care. In the first few months, however, patients used our walk-in service almost exclusively.

Our euphoria was somewhat dampened that first summer when it became necessary for me to fire another staff member—a popular Puerto Rican teacher. This time I was a little better prepared for the community's reaction.

For eight days we had pickets outside Bathgate, although only one of our own staff joined the pickets. All the same, work was disrupted and I was very concerned. (I still had not recovered from the earlier firing of the nurse.) Although firings were few, they took a tremendous toll, both on those being fired and those who did the firing. It was really the worst part of my job.

## CLOUDS ON THE HORIZON

By mid fall of that year certain problems began to surface. Our goal of developing a health plan for each family, and discussing it with them, proved extremely difficult. In many cases, when all the problems were spelled out, it was clearly beyond our capabilities to develop a comprehensive strategy. We also were having trouble involving the families in the planning. The lawyers were appalled at the paternalistic tone taken by the medical staff, which, they pointed out, increased the dependency feelings of the families. They were always saying, "What does the *family* want?"

Another problem was charts. Already the family charts were bulky. It was difficult to look through them quickly to get information. The training of the doctors came out here when we found they were not reading other team members' notes. How to organize a chart so that one could easily communicate through writing became a growing concern.

There were also problems around the team. Physicians continued to dominate the weekly team conference. The nurses didn't know how to handle their new role as team leaders. The family health workers tended to be quiet at the weekly team meetings, except when they were called on. The teams were using George Silver's format for reviewing families, but they didn't really know how to do it. The mechanics of defining the problem, following through, and reporting back to the team had never been worked out. On the average only two families were reviewed at a team conference. And no one was getting his work finished.

The family health worker's role remained a center of controversy. Their training, which had started out in such disastrous fashion, had become quite effective under the aegis of the training department. They were getting excellent nursing training from the Sisters of the Sick Poor, and they were being trained at a fairly sophisticated level by the lawyers on our staff. But as team members they were often perceived as little more than messengers or low-level aides, and their newly acquired skills were not utilized.

The nurses' training as practitioners was haphazard at best. It amounted to no more than three hours a week, with only the pediatricians becoming involved. As far as the nurses' supervisory responsibility and their team leadership role, they received no training. Indeed, at that time we didn't know such training was needed or was even available.

The physicians, trained in the authoritarian hospital setting to work in solo practice and to expect obedience from nurses and other health workers, found it very difficult to treat other team members as colleagues—however good their intentions might be. Their training, like the nurses, had in no way prepared them for effective team leadership or team membership roles.

Yet despite my sense of keen disappointment, there were times when the teams really worked, as these notes from my journal suggest.

> With all our problems, when a team functions well we are confirmed in our belief that this is indeed the best way to help our families. Take the case of the R. family:
>
> A 34-year-old Spanish-speaking man comes into the health center and asks for a doctor to see his wife at home. This is impossible; we have physician staff only to cover the health center. A family health worker, K. Estrada, makes the home visit. She reports a 28-year-old woman looking sick, has sore swollen joints and cannot get out of bed. There is no fever ("otherwise it sounded like rheumatic fever"). We send a vehicle to transport the patient to the center.
>
> An acutely ill woman. Her temperature is now up to 102. It appears to be rheumatic fever. Patient must be hospitalized. She is very upset. What about her children? We try to get a homemaker—no chance for two weeks. A young cousin comes over to act as a homemaker. The father is doing well in a training program. He has a month to go and should not drop out.
>
> The patient is hospitalized. She has rheumatic carditis. She is very unhappy in the hospital; her few visitors and the family health worker are the only persons who speak Spanish. All kinds of tests. Injections. The family health worker finds she is worried about her husband and the young cousin. We finally get a homemaker. But isolation in hospital proves too much and patient signs out of hospital against medical advice.
>
> Home conditions are terrible. The family health worker gets a neighbor to do the shopping. Speaks to husband, encouraging him to stay at work. She fills out a form in English asking for an apartment in the project because of medical disability. (Mother will be partially disabled for six months.)
>
> The nurse visits weekly to give patient injections. The family health worker visits three times weekly, gets vital signs, weighs patient.
>
> Doctor visits every two weeks or when there is a change in weight or vital signs. We have difficulty restricting salt intake.
>
> In the meantime we get children immunized and arrange for eye surgery for one child who has a squint. This is a reasonably easy problem—all family members are cooperative.
>
> Another family: a 21-year-old woman with three children, two of whom have ended up in hospital malnourished. The mother is "im-

mature," lies in bed all day. Looks depressed. The place is a mess.

Argument in team conference as to whether or not to split up the family. Doctor wants to place children. Family health worker says mother wants to keep children. She will give it a try. She visits three times a week. Gets in nearly every time. After two months she states mother is dressing better. Goes out a little, puts on lipstick. Children gaining weight.

Two weeks later family health worker is very upset. Knocked at door. Children are alone. Mother is not at home. (Report that week of a fire in a home where three children who had been left unattended died.) Doctor has a smirk on his face. Family health worker wants to give it another try, but she now admits she is no longer hopeful of keeping the family together.

Family health workers are proving very effective in several areas. Patients discharged from state hospital doing well. Family health workers beam when they learn their weekly visits are "supportive therapy." Validates their work.

Patients are very timid. They come in, not looking at me, not taking off their coats. I always bring in another chair and shake hands with the patient, introducing myself. Many are surprised and smile with embarrassment.

Without any probing, the problems pour forth. In almost every family there seems to be much for the team to do. I do not understand why the doctors do not use other team members more often. They must feel frustrated trying to deal with the psychosocial problems on their own.

The nurses like the practitioner role. Even with their very limited training in this area, they are developing more confidence. Some sport the doctor's white coat; some wear a stethoscope around the neck, very much like medical house staff. A few even begin to imitate the "chutzpah" style they see in some of their physician counterparts.

A team functions well with a good doctor. He allows experimentation, is willing to support staff. The team cares for its members. Communication is frequent, informal. They respect each other's input. A family health worker finds out a new development from a patient. The doctor is impressed, saying he doubts if the patient would have told him this.

The poorly functioning teams are more concerned with their own roles than with the patient. There are endless arguments about who is in charge, whose responsibility it is to do what.

The flexibility of the physician seems to be the key factor for smooth team functioning.

## BACK TO THE DOCTOR

In that first spring at Bathgate, while we were preparing for the opening of the main center, I became convinced that the doctor was the critical variable in team performance. If our health team delivery system was going to work, I reasoned, we must change the doctor, make him more aware of and responsive to the environmental and sociopsychological issues that affected his patients and his teammates.

Since our main center was going to be late in opening (the date was now set for the beginning of August) and since our new complement of doctors and nurses had been hired as of July 1, perhaps a month-long orientation on the community and its problems would help to sensitize these people and make them more effective in their new team assignments.

The orientation was mostly a disaster. The physicians didn't know what they were getting into. We took them to the Police Department, to the Welfare Department, to various social agencies. They said, "What has this got to do with the practice of medicine?" By the end of the first week, they *had* to see patients. This relieved the pressure, but it was clear that the orientation was not going to solve the doctor problem. Instead it set back our social medicine activities, since the doctors and nurses resented what they felt was an attempt to propagandize them.

But we had other plans, too, for improving the team delivery of health care when the main center opened. Since we had to temporarily close Bathgate to staff the new center, we decided to split up the three health teams then operating in Bathgate and mix old team members with new employees. In this way the teams would have a new beginning in the new center.

We felt it would also be useful to formalize our concept of team roles and team operation. So we held a series of meetings with the staff to inform them of their respective roles and responsibilities. Later this "portrait" was put in writing. It is presented here not as the everyday reality of team functioning but rather the way we wanted the teams to operate.

### PORTRAIT OF A TEAM

> There are two health facilities: The Dr. Martin Luther King, Jr. Health Center, which houses six health teams plus a walk-in unit for patients without appointments, and the Bathgate Health Center, which has two health teams. Two teams, which share, on an alternate basis, treatment rooms and a waiting area, comprise a health unit. The units are staffed by a practical nurse, medical assistants, receptionist-appointment clerks, and a secretary.
>
> The primary health team is responsible for providing comprehensive health care to about 1,500 families in a geographical subsection of the area we service. The team consists of two public health nurses,

six family health workers, an internist, and a pediatrician. Specialized back-up services are provided by a part-time psychiatrist or psychologist, and a half-time midwife. Each team is assigned a health advocate (a new health worker trained by lawyers, health education specialists, and community organizers) and a dentist.

Subspecialty consultation is available at the main center in surgery, orthopedics, ophthalmology, optometry, otolaryngology, speech and hearing, dermatology, and allergy. Back-up subspecialty clinics are used at Montefiore Hospital. Obstetrical delivery and hospitalization are carried out at Montefiore or one of its affiliates. Bronx State Hospital provides psychiatric hospitalization.

Our goal is to avoid a rigid team model, and to encourage the appropriate health worker to respond on the basis of family need. While the family health worker is usually the prime contact with the family, any member of the team may serve in that role. However, patients must first go to primary health team members before being referred for specialty consultation.

As key members of the primary care health team, the roles of public health nurse, family health worker, and physician are briefly outlined below.

*The Public Health Nurse Practitioner*

The public health nurse has three major responsibilities: coordination of family care and of the health team; supervision of three family health workers; and practitioner in primary care in specified areas.

In her role of team *coordinator* she is the pivotal person responsible for pulling together the health care for 750 families, which involves formulating family care plans, making appointments for routine care, and reviewing family records. It is also her job to plan and run team conferences and coordinate team activities with other health and social agencies.

Although she is based in the center, as *supervisor* of three family health workers she often accompanies them on home visits to demonstrate new nursing procedures or to review old ones.

As a *practitioner* she has been trained to do well baby care, normal pre- and post-natal care (except for the initial assessment), and routine adult preventive care (ordering chest X-rays, etc.), as well as some psychiatric crisis management and chronic disease care.

*The Family Health Worker*

The family health worker is a neighborhood resident who has been trained as a generalist in home nursing, health education, and social advocacy skills.

Assisting the nurse and physicians on the team, she performs a routine health and social history as well as a medication check. It is also her job to summarize in a brief written paragraph the major problems affecting each household member as well as the health and social problems of the family as a whole, which then become part of the medical record of that family.

In her nursing role she carries out bedside nursing care for bed-bound patients with chronic illnesses, well baby supervision, diet and medication review, post mental hospitalization follow-up, and post-hospital rehabilitation counseling. She is not yet allowed by law to give injections.

She helps the family make appointments in the health center, and arranges hospitalization. She assists the family in negotiations with landlords, the welfare department, the schools, employment agencies, the Housing Authority, Social Security, the health center, and a variety of other agencies.

As a health educator, she checks apartments and houses for accident hazards and lead paint. She may help a health advocate organize a tenants' council in a building, or teach about family planning, nutrition, and acute health problems.

*Physicians*

Pediatricians and internists work as primary care practitioners and have also been assigned consultant-teacher responsibilities on the health teams.

The internists are responsible for rendering primary care services to adults who appear at the center on an appointment or walk-in basis. Pediatricians are the primary care practitioners for the acutely ill child.

Our portrait of the team and its responsibilities seemed clear to us. But would team members, we asked, be willing and able to carry out their assigned roles?

## SHADOW OF THE EL

On the day the main center opened, people were lined up for two blocks waiting for care—despite our having put our full staff to work. Unlike the sense of euphoria we experienced when Bathgate opened, we felt overwhelmed by the task we faced. The place seemed too big for us; we missed the snug, comfortable quality of Bathgate. We had moved from a staff of about 75 at Bathgate to some 300 people in the new center. Instead of three health teams we now had eight. And suddenly I didn't know anybody. At Bathgate I was on the first floor of a two-story building and regularly went to all the team conferences. Now I was on the fifth floor, removed from the teams. When I attended team conferences, I felt attacked. Everyone was asking: "Why isn't this working? Why isn't that working?"

There always seemed to be major conflicts to deal with; we had not developed the routines we needed; many of our employees were still learning their jobs, they were slow, inefficient; we lacked supervisory capability; we couldn't even keep the building clean. There was a false note between the publicity we were getting and what we saw was really going on.

As patient registration increased, so did our problems. We were having trouble with Washington. The first group in OEO had been against any eligibility determination; they did not wish to divide a neighborhood according to income. But now, with the pioneering group gone, the possibility of having to do a means test had become a reality—against which we fought long, hard, and unsuccessfully.

Worse than that, the future of OEO itself seemed in jeopardy. And with Medicaid cut back, our hopes that the program would become self-sustaining were crushed. It looked like year-to-year funding was something we'd have to live with—spending about two months each year hustling for money.

Beyond our troubles with funding, we could see the environment around us deteriorating daily. Garbage collection was getting worse, fires were becoming epidemic, more and more housing was being abandoned. The problems of addiction and crime had taken on crisis proportions. The teams felt paralyzed in the face of what was happening. How could they practice preventive medicine when people were often without heat or hot water and did not get proper food; when sons and daughters were on drugs, and older people were afraid to leave their apartments because of muggings and other crimes.

Of what use, we asked, was a policy to hire only community residents for our training programs and give them preference for all other job slots if, as soon as they were making more money, they opted to leave the community for better schools, more adequate housing, and safer streets. In effect, MLK was creaming the area of its most effective people who might have worked to improve it if they had stayed.

We had tried to reinforce the concept of community, but in a rapidly decaying urban area it no longer seemed to make sense. Lee Bamberger's vision of organizing a neighborhood around the health center in its fight against poverty now seemed an impossible dream. Our only small successes in organizing had been around specific issues that could be resolved in a brief time span. Then the terrible inertia and apathy that characterized the whole area once again prevailed.

Furthermore, the teams' feelings of impotence in the face of such environmental problems exacerbated the problems they were having among themselves and with the rest of the agency. The research we were doing, which was supposed to generate the data we needed for more efficient operation, wasn't working out. The teams often resented the findings or didn't know how to utilize them. And administration seemed to have the same problems in making use of the data. Our appointment system was breaking down. More and more people were making use of our walk-in services so that in effect we were operating a dual system, with many people never referred to a health team for permanent assignment. Medical records were in disarray; charts were often not available when needed. It was not unusual for patients to have to wait two and three hours to see a practitioner. We began to question the use of health teams to deliver care since a small minority of the patients were actually receiving team care. I wrote in my journal:

> Whenever I go down to see a team in my role as project director, I despair of how they are operating. Sensing this, team members turn on me, blaming their shortcomings on inadequate administrative and back-up support. Then I feel guilty; I begin to wish that somehow the teams would disappear and that it's their fault that I've gone out on a limb as an advocate of teams. Today when a visitor asked me what I thought was the ideal size of a team, I replied, "The smaller the better, one is perfect."

Were we, we began asking, turning into just another outpatient facility, delivering the kind of impersonal, crisis oriented medicine we had set out to provide an alternative to?

I was angry. I wrote:

> The agency has schizophrenic goals. On the one hand, we are supposed to provide a first-rate service and we are measured against the best group practices. On the other hand, we are supposed to do the job with people who are not yet trained, who are still in training. We need a topnotch staff with time for teaching. But there is no time and the staff is inadequate.

The teams themselves were going through a very bad period. The friendliness, the generally relaxed pace of the work at Bathgate had given way to a kind of sullen despair in the face of the enormity of the present task. Doctors, nurses, family health workers, each group seemed to be in its own state of crisis.

The family health workers felt they had no real professional standing; their role was unclear on the team and in the community. While some continued to identify with their clients, others no longer wanted to associate with the bedraggled welfare families, the alcoholics, the addicts. They wished to deal only with the upwardly mobile families. *(Over and over again I learn, to my naïve disillusionment, that the poor are no better than anyone else.)*

The nurses felt overwhelmed with their multiple roles—as coordinators of the health team, as nurse practitioners, and, most of all, as supervisors to family health workers. Generally younger than the family health workers, often less mature, they all wanted a head nurse to help them keep the family health workers in line and assist them in dealing with the doctors.

The doctors had their own problems. It seemed to me that some of them who opted to work at MLK did so because they felt that they really couldn't make it in "a more desirable job." To be successful they should be in a hospital or in private practice. Their insecurity led to greater inflexibility, and this resulted in trying to practice in the old way—not understanding the team, really resisting social input.

Everywhere, it seemed, as I looked around the center, doctors and nurses wanted to practice in the old way. And family health workers, who lacked an "old way," wanted one spelled out for them.

It had been better at Bathgate. I thought of the handmade poster one of the nurses had tacked up outside the conference room there. It read:

> "Every human being is a mystery that must be learned slowly, reverently, with care, tenderness and pain, and is never learned completely."

Had we lost our way, I wondered?

## GAINING PERSPECTIVE

By the spring of 1969 I knew I would have to take some kind of break or I would leave the center for good. I was angry, bitter; nothing seemed to be working. A period of time away, perhaps, would help restore perspective. Before leaving I wrote a proposal for a social medicine house staff program. The doctors' orientation fiasco and the difficulty we had in recruiting the kind of doctor we wanted convinced me that we must have a new kind of physician and he would have to be trained over the long term as a social medicine doctor.

After putting the proposal together, I left for England on a work-study fellowship, with Bill Lloyd, the medical director, taking over as acting project director.

The months away were important ones. As I visited health facilities in Scandinavia, Great Britain, Yugoslavia, I had time to reflect on the problems of health team members. The nurses' training as practitioners clearly needed strengthening and I determined this would be a priority item when I returned. We needed to bring more community people into management positions. If we could get the social medicine internship and residency program going, it would be a decided plus for the center as the teams would then have the part-time services of socially oriented physicians. We would find other ways, too, to strengthen our health teams. For of all the programs I observed in operation, none it seemed to me was as exciting or held greater potential than our health center in the South Bronx.

## THE SEARCH FOR ANSWERS

When I returned in November of 1969 after seven months abroad, the center was being swamped by demands for its services. As acting director, Bill Lloyd had

had the difficult task of guiding the center in a period when registrations had tripled due to our having opened registration to all residents of Health Areas 24 and 26 in the previous March. These newly registered patients made about twelve visits per year to the center, or more than twice the average visit rate in prepaid group practices. Despite additions to staff, everyone was under tremendous pressure from the heavy work load. Internists were often forced to see 15–20 patients during an appointment session, making it impossible to provide the thorough and leisurely care previously available. Public health nurses were still trying unsuccessfully to cope with their multiple responsibilities and their greatly increased case loads. Back in Bathgate days, a family health worker might have a case load of 25 families; now she was likely to have well over a hundred—in some cases, 200. All this had resulted in generally low morale and increasing friction among department heads as well as among health team members. As in Bathgate days, I was surprised and upset by the amount of infighting on staff, some of it no doubt due to my own confusion concerning the nature of the problems and my lack of assertiveness in finding answers.

But even in the face of these heavy problems I was experiencing a new surge of optimism. We would find a first-rate administrator who would be able to pull together the many divergent forces operating in the center. We would strengthen the nurse-practitioner role. We would start training community people for top jobs at MLK. And we would push ahead with the social medicine internship and residency program.

I was lucky about this time to meet Dr. David Kindig, who became our first resident in the new I & R program and played a crucial role in shaping its development. Later on, as medical director at MLK, he also worked out a broad reorganization plan for the center. Shortly after my return, I was able to persuade Dr. Regina McCormack, an internist (formerly an RN) and strong advocate of training nurses in the role of primary care practitioner, to join us for a year and work on the curriculum for the nurses' training. As we moved strongly to bring community people into top management positions in the center, we found two most capable candidates in Sonia Valdes and Deloris Smith.

It was only in the search for administrative assistance that we seemed to run into a wall. I talked to people at American Airlines, IBM, other corporations, but they didn't appear to have the answers I was looking for.

Then late one afternoon in January 1970, I sought advice on my administrative problems from Margaret Mahoney of the Carnegie Foundation, which had funded staff anthropologist Alan Harwood's pioneering ethnographic study of the two health areas that the center serviced. Margaret said, "Why don't you talk with Dick Beckhard—he might be able to help you."

The only thing I knew about Beckhard when we met some time later was that he came from the Sloan School of Management at MIT. A little man, sandy hair, quiet, very low key, he looked like a businessman. For fifteen minutes

I talked about the problems we had at MLK. He listened attentively. Then he began by saying, "Well, this is what is going on, and from this we can predict such, and such, and such, and such," drawing a clear picture of the internal dynamics of the center. My reaction, I remember, was, "Wow, what kind of a guy is this!"

He said what we needed at the center were some organization development skills, which, as he talked, I interpreted to mean some kind of sensitivity or T–group training. While I didn't understand exactly what he meant, I was really impressed with this man. Somehow, I felt, we must get his help.

Not too many months after this, he was able to rearrange his incredibly tight schedule to spend some time at the center with me. Over three or four meetings we evolved a relationship. Later I met Irv Rubin, who worked with Beckhard and was also from MIT. Soon after it was decided that Dick would work with the top team while Irv worked with the health care teams, starting with a pilot study of two of the eight.

## ORGANIZATIONAL DEVELOPMENT AT WORK

As the top group met with Beckhard in the early months of 1971, I began to sense some basic changes in attitude taking place–including my own. For one thing, problems were being brought out in the open, possible solutions discussed, and action plans formulated. As we worked with him, I began to get a whole new sense of what it meant to be on a team. I had talked health teams, I had written articles on health teams, I had made speeches on health teams, but I had never really understood that a team was anything more than a group of people who had been labeled a team, each doing his or her respective tasks. The concept of teamwork in the sense of a football team or a basketball team–of each person's performance depending on the performance of other members of the team–had never been really clear to me.

Now it seemed naïve to have thought that we could bring together a highly diverse group of people and expect them to function as a team simply because they had been designated as such. That there were specific team membership and team leadership skills which could be learned was another new idea for me. The fields of organizational psychology, organizational development, group dynamics–none of which the medical student is exposed to in his traditional training–seemed to hold the answers to many of the complex problems that had been besieging us at the center.

For myself, these months working with Beckhard and the top team were a period of clarification of goals–both the center's and my own. I felt MLK should be more involved with educating the community, with training new health teams, in fact setting up a school for health teams. Other top management members felt that a period of consolidation was needed, that the focus should be on making the present patient care system operate more efficiently, of implementing the reorganization plan that had been worked out with the center staff and Beckhard.

I discussed this with Beckhard and with the top group. They were basically opposed to my position. Should I press ahead anyway?

In early 1968 I had written in my journal:

> Administration does not suit me. I bring my work home with me. Often I sit glassy-eyed at dinner, the meal an intrusion between reading letters, memos, drafts, making phone calls. The phone calls are a good indicator of my anxieties. Sometimes for several hours I call a variety of people. Discussing problems. Getting advice. I call George Silver very often, especially when the going gets hot. He helps me clarify the issues and I am less anxious.

The message was there: *administration does not suit me.*

In the Spring of 1971, after a day-long session with the MLK staff, I told Bill Lloyd that I had decided to resign from the center and move over full time to the internship and residency program in social medicine at Montefiore. Bill, with his experience as medical director and acting project director at MLK, was the logical person to take over my administrative duties. Beyond this, we shared the goal of turning over, as soon as possible, the management of MLK to neighborhood people. I knew he would continue to do all that he could to help them develop the requisite management capability.

Assured of the support of the staff and Advisory Board, Bill agreed to stay with the project as its director. I would continue working closely with him and MLK but without the time-consuming responsibilities of heading up the project. In my new position I would have more time for teaching, for developing the school for health teams, and for clinical practice.

Since that day in July 1971 when I left the center, I have kept in close contact with MLK and the continuing struggle to implement the organization development concepts that Beckhard and Rubin have helped us to understand. The center's reorganization, which started when Dave Kindig was medical director, has proceeded under the able and energetic guidance of the new director of health services, Dr. Edward Martin (who also came out of the internship and residency program) and, of course Bill Lloyd, who is the last of the original top group remaining at the center.

If this personal account of the center's evolution has set the stage for what is to follow, I will have accomplished my objective. For this book is primarily concerned with the concrete action steps that MLK has taken to improve the team delivery of health services to the community it serves.

No one involved in this project considers it "the last word" on health teams or team development, Rather, we like to think of this as an interim report on work in progress which will continue indefinitely as health teams evolve along with the institutions that support them.

## NOTES

1. That little has changed in the emergency room at Morrisania in the last six years is made clear by Dr. Steven McCloy's account of his own experiences while on rotation at Morrisania in 1972. See E.R. Diary," by Steven G. McCloy, M.D., *Germinal Ideas,* Vol. 2, No. 3, Internship and Residency Program in Social Medicine, Montefiore Hospital, Bronx, N.Y.
2. G. James, former N.Y.C. Commissioner of Health, in a statement to *The New York Times,* January 27, 1966.
3. Members of the core group (besides me) were William B. Lloyd, medical director; Stella Zahn, head of training; Roy Kurahara, community organization; Jack Schneider, administration; Ron Brooke, research; and Harriet Bograd, lawyer.
4. George A. Silver, M.D. *Family Medical Care–A Report on the Family Health Maintenance Demonstration:* Cambridge, Mass.: Harvard University Press, 1963.

## About Chapter Two

*How do OD consultants actually work? What exactly do they do to help a team function more effectively? Are they involved with sensitivity training and is that some kind of brain washing? Will the team training they're offering be voluntary or is it in fact mandatory? How much time will it take away from the center's real work? And who's paying for this anyway–MIT consultants aren't donating their services?*

*These were some of the questions blowing in the wind when MLK team members assembled at 1:00 PM on a Wednesday afternoon in January 1971 to get their first look at the MIT consultants and hear what they had to say.*

*It's unlikely that anyone attending that meeting remembers much about the words that were spoken. Besides a language barrier (OD has its own jargon problem), experiential training is hard to describe–since experiencing is the thing, not talking about it. Still, team members could get a sense that these people wanted to help, that they thought they could help, that they had done similar training with many other groups, and that, who knows, maybe they did have some answers that would be useful to MLK. While not everyone wanted to buy in that day, some of the teams felt it was at least worth a try.*

*And so the pilot project came into being.*

*Chapter Two tells the consultants' story of how they worked with the teams. Their four-phase approach–data collection, feedback, action planning and evaluation–is seen in action. Also described are some of the tasks or exercises used to help team members increase their group leadership and group membership skills as well as to enhance their overall sense of team.*

*The outcome? Did the fifteen hours spent with the consultants make a real difference? Did the training work? The answer is yes, as a beginning; no as a final solution. The authors, cautiously optimistic, point to further steps required if the effective team delivery of health care is to be fully realized.*

# Chapter Two

# Working with the Primary Care Team: The First Intervention *

*Ronald E. Fry, Bernard A. Lech and Irwin Rubin*

Two bodies of knowledge—organizational psychology and organizational development—were used in the design and implementation of the strategies, interventions, and activities that comprised the MIT pilot program for team improvement at the Dr. Martin Luther King Jr. Health Center in the South Bronx.

Put briefly, organizational psychology provided us with a theoretical framework for dealing with groups and individuals within the organizational setting.[1] Organizational development (OD), which is the application side of organizational psychology, provided us with a set of educational strategies and methods, emphasizing experiential learning.[2]

In this chapter we describe our experiences with two of MLK's eight health care teams, each of which we worked with for some fifteen hours over a period of five weeks. As a first step, it was necessary for us to examine or diagnose the environment in which the health teams operated. To do this, we needed a framework within which to proceed.

## AUTOTHERAPEUTIC MODEL

The conceptual framework we used to help guide us in our work with the health teams consisted of an autotherapeutic or self-renewing model, which is shown in Figure 2–1. The basic assumption underlying this framework is that the environment in which the teams operate inevitably produces uncertainty, anxiety, and frustration. Unless team members can effectively manage these negatives, they will be caught in a downward spiral, which will lead to more anxiety and poorer performance on the job. If, however, they are able to manage the situation effectively, the result will be less anxiety and improved health care delivery.

We call the environment in which a team operates its "life space,"

*
Portions of this chapter were abridged from an unpublished Masters Thesis at the MIT Sloan School of Management, R.E. Fry and B.A. Lech, June 1971.

**Figure 2–1.** The Health Team as an Autotherapeutic Organism

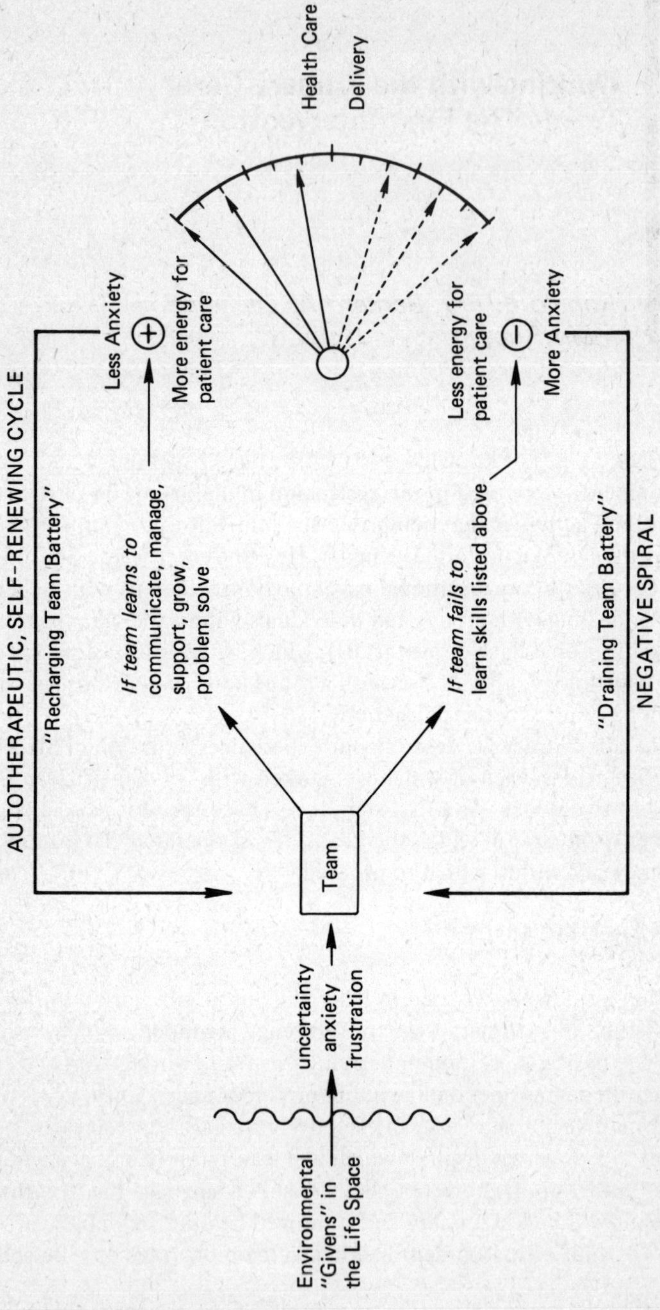

which is shown in Figure 2–2. Many aspects of this life space are slow, difficult, or impossible for the health teams to change. For example, nothing the teams can do is likely to have much effect on the city bureaucracy or the ghetto neighborhood within which the teams must operate.

We might say that the team's job is to manage its interface with this life space. "Manage" as used here means that the team must be able to handle conflict; work out relationships between doctors, nurses, family health workers, etc.; socialize new members; and make decisions so as to effectively cope with and solve the social-medical problems presented by the life space.

Our thesis is that if the teams communicate, support their members, problem solve, etc., the result will be autotherapeutic or self-renewing, like recharging the "team battery" (the upper loop in Figure 2–1). But if team members fail to communicate, support, etc., we believe they will experience more

**Figure 2–2.** The Life Space of a Health Team

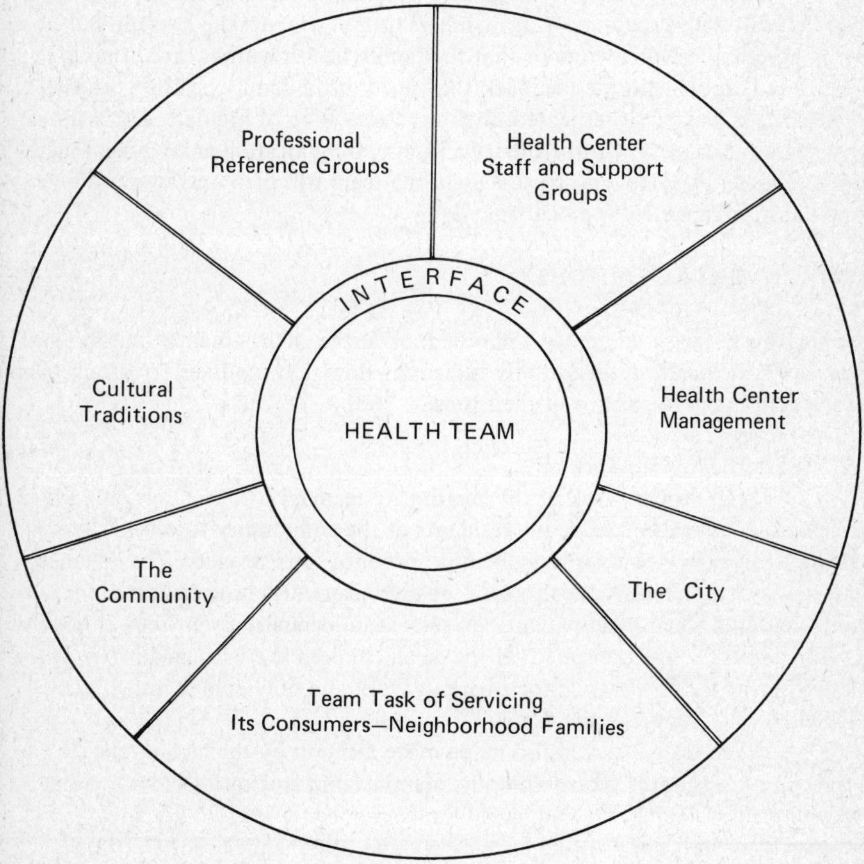

anxiety, which will drain team energy and spirit; in other words, they will be caught in the negative spiral or lower loop in our diagram.[3]

Now let us briefly step through the model. The environment—slow and difficult to change as it is—generates the frustratingly heavy workloads and uncertainty about work priorities. Team members may ask any of the following questions:

> **Doctor**: "Can I get enough valid information from the family health worker about this family's situation to be sure my medical prescription will help?"
> **Public Health Nurse**: "Can I really function as a nurse-practitioner when my training has taught me to follow doctors' orders and ask no questions?"
> **Family Health Worker**: "Do I really know enough to be able to give the doctors and nurses the information they need?"

The anxiety, uncertainty, and frustration reflected in such questions must be dealt with *by the team.* If members do not support the nurse in her new role, if communication is so poor that the family health worker cannot provide doctors and nurses with the feedback they need, if the family health worker does not feel she is trusted or respected, then the lower loop of Figure 2–1 will operate to increase the anxiety. On the other hand, if communication among team members is sufficiently good, and trust is high, the team will then operate on the upper, autotherapeutic loop of Figure 2–1.

## ENVIRONMENTAL FACTORS

Keeping this model in mind, we will now look at the environmental factors that impinge on the health teams, briefly indicating how they are likely to affect team members in the performance of their jobs.

### The Team's Task

The primary task of the health care team is to deliver comprehensive, family-centered health care to the residents of the community it serves.[4] Any task stated in such global terms is likely to produce some anxiety. For instance, what does "comprehensive health care" really mean? And how can care be family-centered when most patients are seen as individuals? Even when this is not the case, how is a family defined? If the small children live with an aunt or other relative during the week while their parents work and only come "home" on weekends, who comprises the family?

The team's task is also made more difficult by the lack of clearly defined and measurable goals. While the complex and frustrating environment makes this unavoidable, the ambiguity the team faces tends to dilute any successes that do occur, causing uncertainty and often depression.

Chronic problems with no easy or clear medical solutions are also a specific source of anxiety for health team members. They not only yield few successes but they afford little if any positive feedback or reinforcement from the patients. A family health worker remarked that what made her happiest was "when Mrs. Y stopped by our office to thank us. But people just never seem to do that very much."

Then there is the problem of patient demands. Beyond being asked to respond to the normal health needs of a patient, some patients also "ask the impossible of me," as one family health worker put it. These "impossibles" range from resolving marital problems to doing the grocery shopping. Even if not actually impossible, such tasks at least create many conflicts around what a team member expects his role to be.

Difficulties also arise around team members' expectations of each other. A family health worker, for instance, who has been trained in practical nursing and community development, may be seen as an "errand girl" or "messenger," and hence treated as such by other team members. This can only cause additional frustration and uncertainty about what her job really is.

Often team members are forced to work in relatively new or unknown areas such as a doctor getting involved in social welfare problems, family health workers in psychiatric problems, or a nurse in the supervision of paraprofessionals. Such behavior is generally at odds with the expectations created by prior training and experience. Adjusting to such roles takes time. And worrying about one's qualifications makes it that much more difficult to act confidently.

All these factors contribute to the complexity of the health teams' task of providing comprehensive patient care.

### Ghetto Community

The following are elements of the community which, inherently, create anxieties for the health teams:

1. Inadequate law enforcement threatens the safety of everyone in the neighborhood, including team members.
2. Low level of education and lack of understanding of or appreciation for preventive medicine add to the health teams' task of educating the community in health care, family planning, nutrition, drug rehabilitation, sanitation, etc.
3. Cultural and economic differences often create communication problems. For example, a doctor's prescription which reads, "To be taken three times per day after meals" reflects a white, middle class perspective. Poor people often do not have the luxury of three meals a day.

Seemingly obvious, straightforward solutions like getting the walls painted, getting children in day care centers, or getting a home maker into a household are generally only partial solutions. And even then, implementation of any such social prescription is no simple task. Total success is nearly impossible and clear-cut success is infrequent. Against such odds, team members cannot help but react in frustrating, depressive, critical manners which create anxieties among themselves and in their patients. One family health worker summed it up: "I'm told not to worry about social problems that I can't handle, but then I have to tell the family I can't help them. And that makes me feel lousy."

**The Urban Monster Megalopolis**

The bureaucracy, politics, and staggering demographic enormities of the city engulfing this health center easily conjure up the image of an unwieldy, thick-skinned creature. Insensitive and unresponsive, the creature moves slowly, uncontrollably, down paths that seem to many, including the "little" health team, to lead nowhere. To the health team serving the community's needs, dealing with both city and large private agencies providing welfare, housing, hospitalization, transportation, and law enforcement services is often a time-consuming, frustrating experience.

For example, a family health worker who arranges her schedule so that she can accompany one of her patients to a hospital for treatment not provided by the health center may find herself with the following dilemma: Should she leave the frightened, Spanish-speaking woman in a waiting room with little hope of adequate communication with doctors (the sick woman may flee) so as to see other needy patients or to attend an important team meeting? Or should she scuttle the remainder of her schedule to stay with the woman? The dilemma increases her uncertainty and, hence, her anxiety.

**Cultural Mix of Team Members**

Health care teams are composed of members ranging widely in nationality, color, religion, and social background. Caucasian, Afro-Americans, Europeans, Asians, Puerto Ricans, Americans, Jews, Catholics, Protestants, residents of poor, middle, and upper class urban and suburban neighborhoods, unmarried, married, with children, without children, separated, divorced—all are represented on the teams. While it might be helpful for teams to have nonwhite doctors, nothing the team can do is going to greatly affect the number of Black or Puerto Rican medical students graduating in the next few years.

Formal education of team members ranges from the M.D. degree to less than a high school diploma. And this directly affects the status of team members. Doctors are at the top, nurses are subordinate to doctors, and family health workers, without recognized professional job roles, are still lower. These vast differences produce gaps in communication, understanding, and expectations that may only be closed through long hours of special effort. Yet the pace of the work tends to preclude any such effort being made.

While the differences in skills and experiences are necessary, the anxiety caused by them needs to be managed. It should be a task of the team to find methods to reduce the uncertainties and frustrations that naturally occur from this cultural mix. Ignoring and suppressing this anxiety will only worsen the situation. For example, a family health worker, intimidated by a doctor's higher status and by her own background of subordination, finds it impossible to ask the doctor about terminology she is not familiar with. This inevitably affects her self-confidence when she communicates with her families and tries to implement a plan of action the team has decided upon. And in the end it is the family who suffers.

**Tug-of-War: Community and Team**

The family health worker is supposed to cultivate the skills of questioning, probing; and collecting information that she needs to perform her job effectively. The community, in many instances, is withdrawn, suspicious, and silent. Since she is also a member of that community, she is certain to experience some uncertainty and frustration centered around violation of community norms and her own sense of survival. Sharing information and feelings openly with other team members may be just too threatening—based on her past experiences in the community. For example, should she communicate private, confidential information about a friend of hers who is also a team patient and the subject of a team conference meeting? Should she reveal that the husband is not living with the family so that his wife and children can enjoy the relative comfort of an apartment in a new housing project which is made possible by Aid for Dependent Children welfare payments? Such a disclosure, she knows, could result in the family's eviction. Unless the resulting anxiety, in addition to the specific problem, is dealt with, the situation can only worsen.

The team approach to health care may require that the long-standing tradition of privacy between doctor and patient be expanded to a team-patient relationship. However, for most team members the tendency is to revert to the established medical model: labeling, diagnosing, and prescribing "in one's head" with only the result shared.

**MLK Management**

Finally, the health center's management is an important aspect of the health teams' life space. It affects the teams in many ways. Our observations suggested that the interaction between health teams and management did not, on the whole, improve the delivery of patient care. Sometimes quite the reverse.

Briefly, the center's organization structure was patterned along traditional hospital lines, with a top-down chain of command. This meant the health delivery teams fell at the bottom of the structure and were, more often than not, the passive recipients of decisions made at the top of the hierarchy, with the latter often lacking the information required to be really responsive to the needs of the teams.

The reporting system also tended to work against facilitating a team operation. As in hospitals, pediatricians reported to a chief of pediatrics, internists to a chief of internal medicine, nurses to a chief of nursing, etc. This had the effect of drawing people outside the team and lessening the cohesive factors. What we encountered in many instances was a group of individuals each doing his or her own tasks independently of other so-called team members. It was a team in name only.

These then were the major factors making up the environment or life space of the health teams over which members had relatively little control. We now will look at the area of greatest potential control—the team's management of itself. It is here that we, as consultants, planned to focus our efforts to help the teams help themselves.

## THE PROCESS FACTORS

To understand how any group manages itself, it is necessary to look at the group's processes—that is, how it goes about doing its work. For instance, how are decisions made? Do people listen to each other? Do most members participate in discussions or do a few consistently dominate? These and other process factors tell us how the group operates, how it goes about doing its tasks.[5]

To evaluate the health teams' managerial effectiveness, we looked at six key process variables, which are critical in all groups: (a) goals or mission, (b) role expectations, (c) decision making, (d) communication/leadership, (e) norms, and (f) conflict management.

It is important to note that all these factors are amenable to change. While the elements of the life space of the teams are slow to change, how a team *manages* its life space is assumed to be subject to change through learning. The key, then, in striving for the autotherapeutic ideal is that the team learn to manage its life space effectively. We will now look at how the teams dealt with each of the process factors listed above.

### Goals or Mission

Any team or group has a purpose. A reason or reasons exist for the formation of the group in the first place. Questions relating to goals are (a) Who sets the goals and how clearly are they defined? (b) How much agreement is there among members concerning the goals? How much commitment? (c) How clearly measurable is goal achievement? (d) How do group goals relate to broader organizational goals? To personal goals?

As we have already seen, members of the MLK health teams experienced considerable uncertainty over their global mission of attempting to provide comprehensive, family-centered health care. Anxiety was also generated because teams did not really know when and if they were succeeding. Questions of priorities and time allocations were also complicated; how does one decide between competing activities in the absence of clearly defined goals? These were some of the unresolved problems relating to goals that the teams needed to work on.

**Role Expectations**

Multiple role expectations is another critical factor affecting members of most groups. Each person, in effect, has a set of expectations of how each of the other members should behave as the group works to achieve its goals. In any group, therefore, there are questions about: (a) the extent to which such expectations are clearly defined and communicated (role ambiguity); (b) the extent to which such expectations are compatible or in conflict (role conflict); (c) the extent to which any individual is capable of meeting these multiple expectations (role overload).

In the two teams we worked with there was little discussion as to what one's job responsibilities really were. Even where a role was clear, it was often not accepted by all team members or not utilized properly. A nurse remarked, "I'm supposed to supervise but I don't have any power to do anything if I find something is wrong." A doctor remarked that he "wished nurses could do more nursing, but they have too many other things to do." Family health workers, perhaps more than any other team members, were not used adequately and their roles were not clear. While they were told they were the team "experts" on the community, more often than not their opinions were not solicited.

Such frustrations and uncertainties result from and reinforce unclear goals and priorities for the total team: "The patient is No. 1." "Medical problems are No. 1." "Social problems are my main concern." "We have to change the community before we can provide comprehensive health care." These differences were rarely discussed; rather, for the most part they were ignored.

A team member's failure to communicate his feelings about what he thinks others expect of him, about what he'd like to do, and about what he feels he has to do results in uncertainty for both himself and the rest of the team. Conflicts and dilemmas that could be dealt with if they were allowed to surface are instead submerged; only the frustration surfaces. The level of concern now becomes "how to cover up what I really feel in order to avoid a fight or argument that I will probably lose." The assumption is that by avoiding such interactions, the team will have more time to perform its task in the community.

Actually, the opposite is true. Energy that might have been expended on the task instead goes into these elaborate cover-ups of feelings. And since any discussion of such problems is avoided, nothing gets resolved.

A nurse remarks that she feels like a "juggler with too many balls." Another says, "I can't keep my head above water." Instead of being in a position to deal with the unavoidable anxieties caused by the environment, the team adds to its frustration, depression and uncertainty by ineffective management of its own processes. By not spending the time required to achieve common goals and clear roles, the resulting anxiety actually interferes with the team's providing effective health care.

**Decision Making**

A group is a problem solving, decision making mechanism. By this we do not mean to imply that an entire group must make all the decisions as a group. The issue is one of relevance and appropriateness: Who has the relevant information and who will have to implement the decision? A group can choose from a range of decision making mechanisms, including decision by default (lack of response), unilateral decision (authority rule), majority vote, consensus, or unanimity.[6]

Any of these forms may be appropriate under certain conditions. And each will have different consequences both in terms of the amount of information available for use in making the decision and the subsequent commitment of members to implement it.

Probably the most obvious requirement in attempting to deal effectively with the South Bronx community and its patients is the need for many different inputs into the decision making process. While some purely medical problems can be resolved unilaterally by the physician, more often the nature of the task dictates that many skills and resources will be needed to diagnose and treat complex social-medical problems. Furthermore, all team members must be commited to team decisions if those decisions are to be effectively implemented. But such commitment, we know, is rarely forthcoming unless all members have participated in the decision making process.

The decision making we observed most frequently on the teams could be characterized as being made by a minority, with most team members noncommittal. Decisions by majority vote and unanimity were not seen at all. Consensus was often solicited, but usually had to be assumed from silence. This kind of decision making is best understood as the "plop effect." At first glance, this hardly seems a method at all, but its invisibility belies its power. When a team member suggests an idea, the result is no response at all, and then another member suggests a new idea. The first member's suggestion has "plopped" without as much as a single response concerning its merits or disadvantages.

Another member, seeing his first "plop," may think, "if that is what happens to his ideas, I won't stick my neck out." The effect spreads until only the most outspoken members offer their ideas. They become the minority making the decisions. While they may sense some uncertainty as to the degree they are supported by others or as to their authority, in the face of an environment that demands action they forge ahead, often railroading a decision through. Such decisions not only limit participation but, even more detrimental, severely reduce commitment to the decisions.

Majority vote and true consensus seem most appropriate in terms of sharing ideas and feedback among all those who should be involved. This puts great emphasis on effective communication: Necessary information and feelings *must* be shared if the team is to manage the anxiety and frustration caused by the environment. The less sharing of such information, the more anxiety is created.

What we observed was little sharing and much anxiety.

**Communication Patterns/Leadership**

If, indeed, a group is a problem solving, decision making mechanism, then the effective flow of information is central to its functioning. Anything that acts to inhibit the flow of information will detract from the group's effectiveness.

A range of factors affects information flow. At a very simple level there are architectural and geographical issues. Meeting space can be designed to facilitate or hinder the flow of communication. Geographically separated facilities may be a barrier to rapid information exchange.

Numerous more subtle factors also exist. Participation—frequency, order, and content—may follow formal lines of authority or status. High status members may speak first, most often, and most convincingly on all issues. The best sources of information needed to solve a problem will, however, vary with the problem. Patterns of communication based exclusively on formal lines of status will not meet many of the group's information needs. The degree to which people feel free to participate, to challenge, to express opinions also significantly affects information flow.

Very much related to the processes of decision making and communication is the area of leadership. To function effectively a group needs many acts of leadership rather than one leader. People often misinterpret such a statement to mean "good groups are leaderless." But this is not what we mean. Rather, depending on the situation and the problem to be solved, different people can and should assume leadership. For instance, the formal leader of a group may defend the organization's official position on a particular issue. Another member may express sharp disagreement and a third may provide help in clarifying the disagreement. This would be an example of some useful acts of leadership. We repeat: It is highly unlikely that in any group there will be one person capable of meeting all of a group's leadership needs.

The communication patterns and leadership we observed on the MLK health teams in general relied on the model team members knew best—in this case, *"follow the doctor."* Acts of leadership by other team members were seldom attempted; and when they were, we saw very little support forthcoming from other members. Several family health workers stated to us (in interviews, not publicly) that since they were closest to the families, they ought to have more of a say in what gets done and how it gets done. These few forceful family health workers either eventually influenced a team decision or "went down swinging," saying " . . . that just won't work with that family!" But they were in the minority, and had little support from the others.

The effect of this traditional model of leadership was decision making by expert medical power, with lack of commitment and support from quiet team members.

### Norm Structure

Norms are the unwritten rules that govern any group. Whether they are understood as such or just "felt," they are powerful determinants of how members will behave. They define what is good or bad, acceptable or unacceptable if one is to be a functioning member of this group. They often take on the quality of laws: "It's the way we do things around here." Their existence is most clear-cut when they are violated—quiet uneasiness, shifting in one's chair, joking reminders are all observable. Repeated violation of norms often leads to psychological or even physical expulsion.

Norms take on particular potency because they influence all of the other areas we have discussed. For instance, the MLK teams we studied exhibited the following powerful norms:

1. In making a decision, "silence means consent."
2. Doctors are more important than other team members—we don't disagree with them; we wait for them to lead.
3. Conflict is dangerous, both task conflicts and interpersonal disagreements—"it's best to let sleeping dogs lie."
4. Positive feelings, praise, support are not shared—"we're all professionals here to do a job" (as if professionals were not people).
5. The difficulties inherent in our task preclude the possibility of our being flexible in respect to our own internal group processes.

The effect of these norms, and others like them, is to guarantee that a team gets caught in a negative spiral. The task demands flexibility; the teams are inflexible. The task underscores the need for some place to recharge one's emotional battery; the team does not provide this opportunity. The task demands maximum flow of information and frequent decisions by consensus; but team members are reluctant to share ideas and feelings; decisions most often are made by a minority, with other members noncommittal.

The cost of failing to develop norms of flexibility, support, and openness of communication is high indeed. For in addition to precluding these norms, it also precludes the development of a set of higher order or meta norms, which involve developing the capacity to become self-renewing or autotherapeutic. For this to take place, controlled experimentation must be sanctioned, along with risk taking, failure, and evaluation of outcomes. In the absence of norms that support and reinforce these kinds of behaviors, a team will end up fighting two enemies—its task and itself.

**Conflict Management**

Conflict management, although overlapping considerably with other process factors discussed, is important as a separate process factor because it determines whether team members will be able to work together successfully despite their many differences. When we use the term "conflict management," we mean both solving a problem involving disagreeing parties and getting adversary parties to accept and live with their differences without compromising the overall team functioning.

Openness is often the key to successful conflict resolution, regardless of environmental givens. Lawrence and Lorsch lend support here by saying, "In organizations existing in quite different environments, we have found that effective conflict management occurs when individuals deal openly with conflict and work the problem until they reach a resolution which is best in terms of organizational goals."[7]

In the health center we observed few members who allowed conflict to surface as it developed. There appeared to be an implicit norm for smoothing over conflicts, as if to preserve the myth of the perfect team. Several members said, "I keep quiet about what bothers me so it doesn't interfere with daily activities." And although three members of one team each spoke to us in private about the same issue, not one of them permitted the conflict to surface in the team meeting, where it might have been resolved.

While we never observed the direct effects of such buried and smoothed-over conflicts, we were told that such conflicts produced an intolerable buildup of anxiety which eventually resulted in a blowup or personnel turnover. At the very least these conditions must result in a loss of motivation and commitment, with communication seriously impaired within the team. For instance, during our sessions we noted some members consistently avoided others when voluntary subgroups were formed. This behavior, we suspect, was the effect of unexpressed feelings about some past conflict which had not been effectively managed.

But perhaps the most important result of this failure to deal with conflicts is the link between team processes and team members' ability to work with the families they serve, particularly family health workers, who are supposed to constructively intervene into family conflicts. Unwillingness to risk surfacing such conflicts within the team and deal with them is likely to be reflected in sidestepping family conflicts. Such avoidance also deprives team members of the opportunity to practice and develop intervention skills. While the immediate result of sidestepping is relatively painless, ultimately the price is increased anxiety and ineffectiveness in helping the patient-families.

Family-centered comprehensive care requires a team to operate much as a family *that deals with or manages its own problems.* When it has achieved this goal it will be in a far better position to serve neighborhood families.

Before moving to a description of the specific consultant interventions designed to help teams learn to manage their processes more effectively, we will examine the overall consulting model we relied upon in our work.

## THE CONSULTING MODEL

Models give the consultant an organized way of thinking. Instead of responding only on the basis of what "feels good" or "seemed right at the time," conceptual models can help the consultant begin to make thought processes explicit that previously were implicit or uncertain to both consultant and client.

If a consultant finds himself without some reference point—some way of explaining "where he's at"—his uncertainty leads to anxiety, which can be sensed by even the most naïve client. This is likely to lead to an increase in the client's anxiety, which then means that the consultant has made life tougher in terms of readiness for change. One only has to be stopped unexpectedly in a hallway during his first visit to the client system and asked, "What are you going to do on the teams? And have you done this before?" by a person who has only one minute to listen, in order to realize the importance of some consistent model framework, or guidelines. The use of a model—in this case the Kolb-Frohman model for planned change—to which we could relate our perceptions, behavior, and activities proved invaluable to us in the program.

Following is a brief look at the seven phases of the Kolb-Frohman model (see Fig. 2–3) and how we made use of them, with emphasis on a few key learning points we felt were particularly important. This seven-phase Kolb-Frohman model is an elaboration of the basic action research approach, which involves four phases: (1) data collection, (2) summarization and feedback, (3) action planning, and (4) evaluation.

### Scouting, Phase One

Since the entire health center was our first "client system," a way had to be found to enter the total system in order to determine which of the eight health teams wanted to consider working with us. Some of the questions we had to answer were: Can we let the administration choose the teams? Should we work through the formal power structure? What about the inevitable rumors—how will we deal with them?

In a highly interdependent organization with a diffuse power base, we were most concerned with soliciting and sending valid information. This meant dealing directly with the teams as much as possible rather than through the administration. We avoided the assumption that all information from the top of the organization was valid, particularly when it concerned the teams at the lower end of the system. In many cases the right hand really did not know what

**Figure 2–3.** The Kolb-Frohman Model for Planned Change

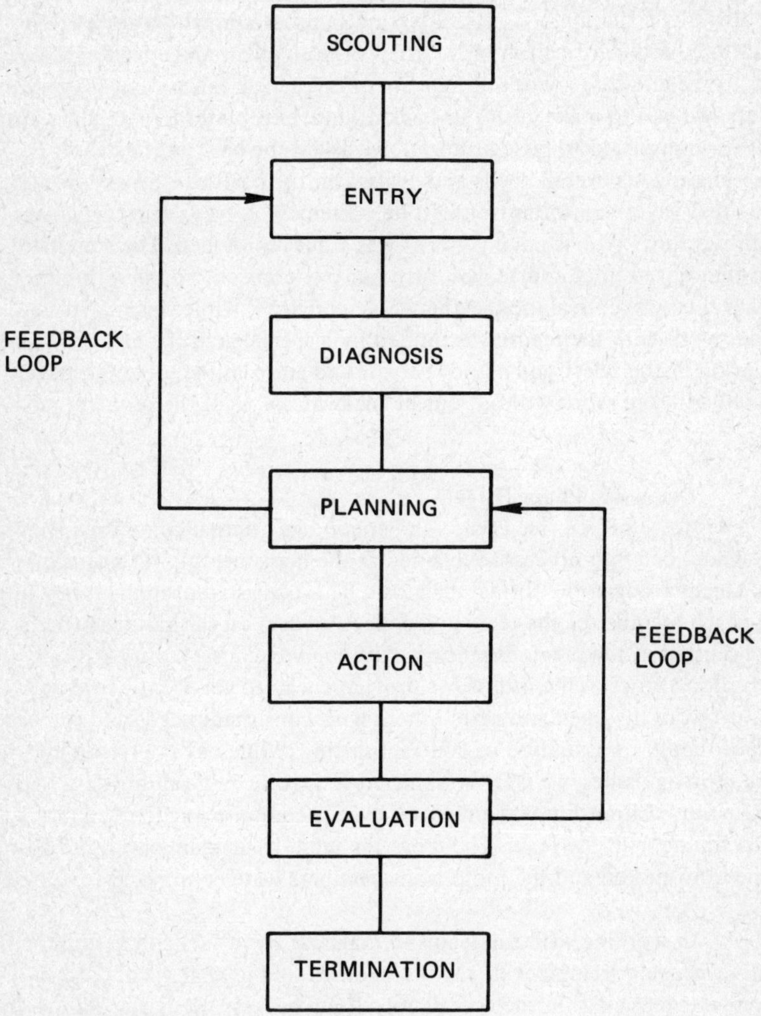


ɔurce: D. Kolb and A. Frohman, "An Organization Development Approach to Consulting," *'oan Management Review* 12:1 (Fall 1970).

the left hand was doing. All this led to our scheduling a mass meeting with the eight teams.

### Entry, Phase Two

The meeting provided a formal introduction to the potential clients. It was also the beginning of contract setting—a process in which perceptions, expectations, and clarification of the roles of both client and consultant are shared, to the end that a working agreement is reached. Since we were very much outsiders, we had to make clear our background, expectations, and goals. And since it was important to be legitimized, we asked the head of the center to introduce us, sharing his overall needs and goals with the health teams and how he thought that we, as consultants, might help them. However, legitimacy can be other things too. "Who is paying you?" was a question asked. The statement behind that question of course was, "If your pay comes from operating funds, we'll take a very skeptical look at the whole activity." While this was not an issue since our work with the teams was funded by a special grant from the Carnegie Foundation, if the question had not been raised and clarified, it could have interfered with our work without our being aware of what the problem really was.

### Diagnosis, Phase Three

To reinforce free choice and encourage internal commitment, we used a shared decision process (explained at the mass meeting) to select the two teams. Then we began the formal diagnosis. This consisted of individually interviewing each member of the team and collecting data on the various process issues discussed in the previous section. Although diagnosis occurs throughout the consulting process, the interviews provide a way to get client needs and resources out in the open and match them with consultant needs and resources. It is a negotiable continuation of contract setting. While our interviews clearly focused on team issues, we were committed to feeding back all the data. An open, trusting relationship was enhanced by our commitment to collaborate on action planning with the team. The more the team became involved, the more valid the information and the more team members were committed to taking action.

In working with the teams to diagnose their data and define their priorities, silence or reluctant or vague responses told us that we needed to rethink our previous stage in the overall consulting process. Remarks like, "I don't know what this meeting was supposed to do for us" indicated that we had not effectively dealt with the contract issues, which meant we needed to go back over our expectations with the teams. In a sense, the contract was really renegotiated at each weekly session by discussing where we had been and where we were going. This also led to a basic change in our overall goals: we moved away from attempting attitude change and decided to try for early successes through structural and behavioral changes. We had misread the teams' level of readiness and were about to push too fast. This also had implications for the future: some quick successes might "unfreeze" team members sufficiently to make them willing to take more risks later on.

**Planning, Phase Four**

The decision to push for some early success experiences affected our planning. It required our using expert power as opposed to trust-based power, which has its own element of risk. However, by (1) sharing our diagnosis of the data with the teams, (2) sharing our design for quick success experiences around improving team conferences, and (3) selecting an activity that all team members recognized as an important and legitimate task, we tried to build a trusting climate. In this way it became less risky to assert our "expertise" and be more directive in planning specific interventions.

But we also had to recognize that increased reliance on us as experts rather than facilitators resulted in increased dependency, which then had to be reduced in the termination stage of the consulting process. Although we tried to design specific actions to make team members aware of their own resources and capabilities, our participation at times overshadowed this objective. Using a consulting model to assist in anticipating such problems helped us. With 20–20 hindsight, it is clear we could have used it more.

**Action, Phase Five**

Whatever actions are taken, whether they result in outright failures or just unanticipated consequences, they only become dysfunctional when the consultant loses sight of his framework, strategy, and contract with the client. When either success or failure–or anything in between–is related back to the diagnosis and to the overall learning goal, it can be helpful to both consultant and client. While dealing with resistance is crucial (sufficiently so to be discussed separately below), we will only emphasize here that client resistance to change at the stage of implementing actions can and should play an expected and helpful role in innovation.[8]

**Evaluation, Phase Six**

The importance of clear, verbalized, shared criteria for evaluation cannot be overemphasized. The team's recognition of a need to develop flexibility led to selecting activities requiring experimentation. Experiments, to be useful, require descriptive evaluation from which team members can learn and grow, not win or lose.

It was important to emphasize personal team ownership of action plans and results. If the teams decided to try something new at a team meeting, we suggested that they take the following actions to insure building the base for internal commitment: decide who was going to carry out an individual task, who was to observe the new behavior or procedure for later evaluation, and when the experiment would be discussed. In this way, team members were more likely to experience a sense of controlling their own processes as opposed to being controlled by the consultants.

In our "where we've been" introduction to each session we evaluated the learning and progress to date. We ended every session with a sharing of observations and evaluations aimed at improving the following week's session. We also began a gradual transfer to the two teams of more and more ownership of planning, evaluating, and follow-up in anticipation of our termination.

### Termination, Phase Seven

Anticipating and planning for termination of the client-consultant activities is a consulting necessity. While a consultant may be attaining great objectives while pushing a team and using his "expert" power, his sudden, casually planned exit can create such anxieties on the team as to negate all his previous efforts. Use of a consulting framework such as the Kolb-Frohman model can help to avoid this and aid in proper planning.

We attempted to consider termination issues such as client dependency throughout our work with the teams. Some of our interventions emphasized the team's ownership of the data. As we have pointed out, we hoped in this way the teams would realize they had the responsibility and the capability to carry on at their own initiative rather than at the consultants.' However, again with hindsight, this was not sufficient. We should have placed greater emphasis on termination beginning with the entry phase and proceeding throughout the entire consulting process.

### Dealing with Client Resistance

How the consultant reads the signals of client resistance is crucial to effective diagnosis. Behavior such as refusal, criticism, silence, etc., should be interpreted as valid information for checking and possibly altering the diagnosis. For example, resistance in the form of apprehension, reluctance or refusal at the implementation phase of the program may indicate the consultant misread the team's readiness in an earlier phase in the consulting process such as contract setting or action planning. Should the consultant react defensively, seem overwhelmed, or be overly saddened, he may increase the very anxiety he is trying to help the team control. He may be implicitly signaling that he cannot handle his client: that the client is in worse shape than either had imagined, or that the consultant's perceived competence is less than the client had anticipated.

If the consultant is to use the client's resistance productively, he must assume that this behavior is the client's way of sending another message as to "where he is at" and thus his readiness for change. By sensing the resistance, determining the underlying message and supporting the feedback, the consultant is also reinforcing one form of effective diagnosis and problem solving: feedback, evaluation, and reduction of anxiety associated with the risk of resisting.

**Summary**

Planned change is enhanced whenever a process can be explicitly described, which is what we have attempted to do here.

It should be emphasized that the seven phases of this model overlap, and that looking back and ahead are appropriate processes in any consulting phase. For instance, data collection and diagnosis is not merely a formal one-shot process; it occurs throughout the client-consultant relationship. Hearing over the public address system the names of doctors, nurses, and family health workers being called to the mass meeting instead of teams being asked to assemble represented informal data gathering which we used to diagnose the state of this complex social system.

The more we understand why we did something that "felt good" at the time, the more we can teach and transfer the skills of planned change to others, thereby improving the health of the group, organization, system, or society within which we are working. Had we to do it over again, we would put even greater emphasis on learning about the consulting process throughout the program. The results are helpful to both client and consultant, both immediately and in the longer run.

We will now describe some of the interventions we used in helping the teams unfreeze.

## CONSULTANT INTERVENTIONS

Intervention has been defined as a direct attempt to influence the ongoing behavior of organizations by coming between or among persons, groups, or subsystems. In the broad sense, everything the consultant does (or does not do), *including* the establishment of the relationship between consultant and client, is an intervention. And *what* he does may range from observing a group of people at work and commenting on their process to asking them to perform specific tasks, the goal of which is experiential learning.

Our initial activity with the teams, as we have already stated, was to interview each member individually, using both open-ended questions, as shown in Table 2–1, and a team interaction form, which is shown in Table 2–2. We explained at the beginning of the interview that many of the team members' remarks would be anonymously fed back to the entire team. As might be expected, the data from the interviews showed many problem areas. There were concerns about team goals, individual roles, relations with the rest of the agency,

**Table 2–1. Interview Agenda**

Name____________________________

Team____________________________

A. Contract setting issues
   1. note taking
   2. confidentiality–data will be fed back anonymously
   3. check back at end of interview on what has been written down

B. Perception of own role/job
   1. what, how, with whom

C. What could other team members do to make you more productive/satisfied?

D. What do other team members do which makes your job more difficult and less satisfying?

E. Team's major strengths and weaknesses

F. Weekly staff meetings–how useful/what could make them better?

G. Kinds of decisions team does/should make as a team
   1. what constitutes a "crisis" for this team?

H. Fill out team interaction form

interpersonal conflicts, and so on. After we had categorized and summarized all this material, we fed back the data at our first meeting with the team as a whole. (See Table 2–3 for data summary.)

Team members' reactions to the data presented during the feedback session were varied. For some, the result was one of surprise–"I didn't realize people felt that way about this team!" Others had been unaware that many of their own concerns were widely shared by other members of the team. Before the feedback session, many people believed that they were the only ones experiencing certain difficulties. The most frequent reaction could be characterized as: "These problems have been around–*under the surface*–for a long time. Now they have been collected, summarized, and are out on the table for all of us to see."

In other words, the teams were provided with an image or picture of their present state based on information collected from the most valid sources available–the team members themselves. As a result of the interview-feedback

**Table 2–2. Team Interaction Form**

| | | |
|---|---|---|
| A. *Communication* | | |
| I often feel as if no one really listens to anyone else | 1 2 3 4 5 6 7 | People really listen to one another's ideas and points of view |
| I often feel hesitant to speak up in team meetings | 1 2 3 4 5 6 7 | I feel free to speak up in team meetings |
| B. *Teamwork* | | |
| Around here it's everyone for himself–we really operate as separate individuals | 1 2 3 4 5 6 7 | Everyone pulls together–we really support and help one another |
| C. *Team Management* | | |
| A few individuals really make most of the decisions on this team | 1 2 3 4 5 6 7 | We all contribute to the decisions made by this team |
| Disagreements are ignored or avoided on this team | 1 2 3 4 5 6 7 | We deal directly and openly with disagreements on this team |
| I often feel I have more to contribute to this team than others seem to recognize | 1 2 3 4 5 6 7 | I really feel as if others recognize the many contributions I can make on this team |
| I often feel as if I have no power/influence over what happens on this team | 1 2 3 4 5 6 7 | I really feel as if I can influence what happens on this team |

process, teams owned the information and shared the image of their present state. This shared ownership helped to create a heightened desire and commitment on the part of team members to solve their own problems. Now we could go on to help them set priorities for the multiple issues reflected in their data; generate alternative solutions to the problems identified; and develop a clear

**Table 2–3. Summary Feedback of Interview Results**

The following suggests one way of feeding back a large conglomeration of remarks so as to help a team begin to set priorities for issues it feels are relevant. The examples here were collected from both teams, with names omitted to preserve anonymity.

A. *How Work Gets Done*

1. Team goals; examples:
   - (a) we react to crises rather than planning
   - (b) we never have decided on what team should be doing: we *should*
   - (c) differing priorities; teaching, medical, social, build agency
   - (d) very little time for joint planning with nurse for patient/family

2. Individual roles/responsibilities; examples:
   - (a) FHWs not adequately utilized, roles not clear; should feel it is her patient
   - (b) nurses should do more medical and delegate more to FHWs
   - (c) team coordinator should be more of an administrator and not concerned primarily with medical care
   - (d) follow-up weak
   - (e) our roles should be better defined
   - (f) you can't ask someone for something if it's not their job

3. Decision making; examples:
   - (a) we should never decide what a family should do without them involved, except for absolute medical problems
   - (b) we should spend some time assessing how the team is doing
   - (c) decisions should be made only by people involved
   - (d) FHWs are closest to patients and *ought* to have more to say about what gets done, how, etc.

4. Relations with other groups/rest of agency; examples:
   - (a) I'm worried about this place, no managers and no goals
   - (b) arbitrary decisions handed down from top don't help
   - (c) no real autonomy as a team, no control over budget; many of us are responsible to bosses outside the team
   - (d) no ability to choose our own staff

B. *What It Feels Like to Work Around Here*

1. Praise, support, feedback; examples:
   - (a) more praise, support would help us cope with crises/mundane tasks
   - (b) we should appreciate each other's pressures
   - (c) little credit/respect given for a job well done
   - (d) you can really trust some people to do a job—this is very satisfying

**Table 2–3. (cont.)**

2. Individual worth and contribution; examples:
   (a) FHWs used to speak up; now we won't buck the nurse or Dr.; we've been put down and have given up fighting back
   (b) lots of roles dumped on nurses; FHWs may feel at "end of the line"
   (c) often made to feel untrusted/inadequate in my job
   (d) my opinion not as valued as the "authority"
   (e) people always checking up

3. Pace and sense of accomplishment; examples:
   (a) around here everything pulls you down, there is nothing pulling you up
   (b) this job is an ongoing crisis
   (c) the work day never seems to end
   (d) environment problems seem to have no solutions

C. *Interpersonal*

1. Communication style; examples:
   (a) some doctors should try to check with nurse more
   (b) I feel bad when someone else deals with my patient and we haven't arranged to swap patients

2. Communication frequency; examples:
   (a) some people talk too much, others talk too little
   (b) one team member not keen on lab report put on desk by another without instructions
   (c) one team member makes me feel stupid so I don't ask questions anymore.

3. Interpersonal conflicts; examples:
   (a) personality frictions have to be resolved; we should cultivate individual strengths instead of ignoring personal conflicts
   (b) one team member is sometimes too harsh in judgment when a task isn't done—sometimes people just plain forget or make mistakes

D. *Issues Outside the Team*

1. There are too many problems we have no control over, that seem to have no solutions (lead paint, lousy police protection, rats, drugs, welfare, psychological problems in families, alcoholism).
2. Lab, X-ray work, and getting records often slow.
3. We have no ability to choose our own staff.
4. We are just too crowded together.
5. We have no real autonomy as a team, no control over budget.
6. Lots of research but no implementation and no benefit to us.

**Table 2–3. (cont.)**

7. Arbitrary decisions at the top are based on whims, not reason.
8. I can't get any satisfaction bucking welfare and having to tell family I can't help them.
9. You can't expect to have an efficient team in a sloppy organization.

E. *Team Conference Issues*

1. Mechanism:
   (a) minutes help, rotating chairmanship is good
   (b) conferences are only good when we present a problem, work on a solution, try the solution and then review the results
   (c) always FHW who presents a family case; doctors and nurses should too; "implies" doctors and nurses are not concerned about families
   (d) they are sometimes all talk and no action
   (e) time-keeping and agenda are important
   (f) rotating leader not good

2. Objectives:
   (a) should be a place to learn from each other
   (b) should be able to develop plans of action but there is little goal setting or agenda setting
   (c) we need to focus on common, solvable problems; we waste too much time on impossible social problems
   (d) it is useful to get together as a total team to talk together, develop consensus of all members, get some people to say more, and others to say less
   (e) for the team, they seem to range from great to poor; they are great when something is solved; they are poor when you don't stick to the task; for instance, meeting spent analyzing FHW's role was a poor meeting

3. Participation:
   (a) if everyone gets interested, we can really get at it
   (b) professionals can be overpowering
   (c) conference is not useful for me—I'm in the outer ring
   (d) communication flows well; everyone attends
   (e) push people to do more of their own case summaries
   (f) quiet FHWs have a lot to contribute

---

and shared set of change objectives or goals—an image of what a more ideal or improved state would be.

This data collection-action planning approach that we used in our work with the MLK teams helped us in a number of ways:

1. It enhanced our knowledge of the environment and the team in a short period of time.
2. Through interviewing we began to establish an open, trusting rapport with the team members.
3. Allowing the team to decide what it wanted to work on from the data it generated counteracted the fear that everyone (administration, patients, researchers) only wanted to take from the team and that no one was really interested in helping. By sharing control of the issues to be worked on, we reinforced our goal of helping team members help themselves instead of coming to them with predetermined or hidden agendas.
4. Finally, this approach provided a basic problem solving model where those who are part of the problem are involved in the solution; where information is solicited from the most valid sources—team members themselves; and where alternatives are generated in terms of specific actions, which are then evaluated and either continued, modified, or stopped.

The tasks we asked the teams to work on all related directly to the problems that were apparent in their data. They ranged from the relatively safe task of planning an agenda to a collage exercise, the purpose of which was to get feelings expressed and recognized as a legitimate part of the real work situation. Our role as consultants became more facilitative and somewhat less directive as our relationship continued, although we did exercise leadership and control in specific exercises. In all the assigned tasks our goal was to provide our clients with the opportunity to learn from experiencing directly rather than read about or hear a lecture on a subject, although we also made use of these as helpful reinforcers or backups.

### Focus on Team Meetings

Since we had decided that the teams needed a quick success experience to increase their confidence in what was for them essentially a new approach to learning, and since team members themselves saw this as valid, it was agreed that the initial focus should be on a relatively easy task—improving team meetings.

To achieve this objective, the teams undertook the task of analyzing the data from the interviews that related to team conferences (see section E of Table 2–3 for a summary of team conference issues). They then selected one or two "behavioral prescriptions" to implement at their next conference. The goal was to make that next meeting the "best meeting ever."

Formal "observer" roles were given to volunteers who would evaluate changes in the team conference; on one team formal "helper" roles were also given to volunteers to assist the team conference leader if he or she requested help.

A formal planning procedure was introduced. Each week several team members met a few days prior to the team conference to evaluate feedback from the last meeting and plan an agenda for the next meeting. The resulting "behavioral prescriptions" were structural or procedural: use of a checklist for the conference chairman, giving each person an opportunity to speak, rotating the chairman, passing in evaluation cards or hearing from formal observers at the end of meetings, and trying different types of presentations.

The structural changes provided an opportunity for new inputs from quiet team members. For the first time, in most cases, family health workers became involved in planning; and medical assistants were, for the first time, invited to attend the meetings. Various team members took on new roles (chairman, planner, observer, helper) before the entire team.

Quick improvements–such as a reduction in uncertainty about what the meeting was supposed to be about and the opportunity to become involved with planning a case presentation–generated noticeable interest and eagerness to attend. The team began to observe, evaluate, modify, and reinforce some of its processes.

Some members, however, were reluctant to try the new formal helper and observer roles for fear that their lack of skill and practice would show. They expressed the need for more direction as to what to observe. Therefore, in our sessions with the teams we began devoting time to sharing our observations for the purpose of helping them develop their own observational skills. Also the growing acceptance of a formal observer role gradually lessened the risk for other team members to share ideas and feelings even when they were directed at a particular person. This kind of participation began to be appreciated as helpful to the team since it generated useful and valid information. Anxiety also seemed to be reduced as team members expressed willingness to help and be helped.

**Communication-Feedback Exercise**

To emphasize the importance of open communication and feedback, we devised a communication-feedback exercise that made use of the doctors' power base, since physicians were clearly the most powerful team members. Our goals were to emphasize the usefulness of helpful feedback; reinforce the new norm of experimentation by encouraging individuals to try new styles of behavior; and underscore the importance of sharing valid information. Working together (without consultants present), the doctors devised individual behavioral prescriptions for "improving my communications style."

Some of the prescriptions were:

"I will not be the first one to fill silences."

"I'll listen more and won't clarify or restate unless asked to do so."

"I won't run on over two minutes."

"I'll check when I bring up something new to see if it is relevant."

Each doctor decided to evaluate each other doctor, share their prescriptions with the entire team, invite others to give feedback and to meet briefly after each team conference to check on their progress.

Particularly significant for our team-building efforts was the effect on the nurses and family health workers at seeing doctors experiment with communication and feedback. If the physicians on the team were willing to take risks, to try out new behavioral styles, and to share these experiences with other team members, it must mean that the doctors trusted their teammates and were concerned with overall team functioning. Nondoctors too, they reasoned, could now start to experiment behaviorally and offer feedback to others—tentatively at first but then with growing confidence. Thus the sense of team became enhanced.

Working with the doctors as a group was an example of effective consultant use of an "environmental given," i.e., a professionally and culturally defined subgroup of the team. Using their roles as "image setters" and "givers of power," the doctors began to build the team instead of just controlling it.

**Role Negotiation Process**

To decrease dependence on the consultants and to teach new facilitative skills to team members, one of our interventions involved a role negotiation exercise.[9] The design called for the development of the "third-party facilitator" role on the team to help other team members solve a problem.[10]

As homework, each team member was asked to fill out and sign individual worksheets for all other team members. The signer was asked to briefly state at least one good example of what "you think the team member named at the top of the sheet could do:

1. *more* or *better* in order to help you work more effectively
2. the *same* which is now helping you
3. *less* of in order to help you

These sheets were given to the person whose name appeared at the top prior to the negotiation session.

When the team met with the consultants, two volunteers were asked to negotiate a conflict, using the consultant as the facilitator, with other team members observing. (Such a setup is often called a fishbowl exercise where the "inside" group is doing something while encircled by an "outer" group that is observing the inside group's behavior.) After the demonstration, our plan had been that the other members would pair off with a facilitator and do their own negotiations. However, they were not ready to take the plunge—they needed to ease into this new activity and manage it at their own pace. Some balked at the rigid structure; others said there was not sufficient time, which may have been a way of avoiding what they saw as a risky situation. During the discussion that ensued a team member remarked, "I can't see why we need this procedure to get at problems between us. Wait—I do so. It's because we just don't do it otherwise!"

While we did not push the teams to focus on feelings (in order to minimize the initial risk associated with the new exercise), feelings did come out, and prompted some healthy discussion. Examples of issues were: family health worker to internist: "I felt bad when you said what you did . . . " ; doctor to FHW: "It would help me more if you tried to describe with facts, rather than label with opinions and judgments, the situations you relate to me."

Their sense of ownership of the information on the sheets prompted some team members to say that they would see to it that negotiations took place in the future—at a more convenient time and place. One doctor remarked, "These sheets fascinate me! I'm certainly going to try to see some people about them in the next few weeks."

### Collage Exercise

As we neared the end of our pilot work with the two health teams, we sensed that team members were now ready to deal more explicitly with feelings—if they could be provided with a reasonably safe vehicle for this. We also felt it important to encourage the sharing of feelings about the team and the individual's relationship to the team.

The vehicle we selected to try and get at such feelings was a collage exercise. The homework for this session was to express, on a large sheet of paper, "what it feels like to work on this team," using sketches, words, magazine cut-outs, or any combination of these the team member wished. The sheets were not to be signed.

When we met, the papers were posted around the room and members eagerly viewed the artistic expressions of their fellows. The discussion started with team members volunteering what they thought the picture said or what they thought the person who made the collage was feeling when he or she did it. Before the session ended all members had given their interpretations of the collages. For example, one collage pictured the team as a battery to which members could "hook up and get charged." There was general agreement that to be effective (autotherapeutic) the team needs to recharge the emotional batteries of its members which get drained by the anxiety-producing environment.

An exciting outcome of this exercise was that some team members said they now could see that their difficulty in expressing feelings of frustration, isolation, or inadequacy was really a fear of being seen as weak or unable to cope with the job; but it was *good* to get these feelings out if the person expressing them received help and support in an atmosphere of trust and openness.

### Theory Memos

While our learning strategy obviously stressed the experiential approach, we also used theory inputs at times. The memos we selected we hoped would reinforce, in our absence, the concepts or methods the team had already worked with. This we felt would reduce dependence upon our presence, yet at the same time legitimize us as a source of useful knowledge.

Two short papers on "Group Process" and "Chairmanship" were distributed following our session on behavioral prescriptions for improving team meetings. A subgroup of a team received a "Force-Field" memo to use as a diagnostic tool for a problem they were going to work on. And at the request of some members, an "Observation-Feedback" memo was distributed to the teams after the evaluation session, which concluded our main activities with the teams.

Although it is hard to judge the effectiveness of these memos, we expect that the best read and most used was the one requested by some team members. Here we were responding to a felt need on their part—not an implied or presumed need on our part.

We do know that reactions varied in terms of professional training. Doctors expressed interest in reading the memos. A group of nurses said they could not use the "Force-Field" memo because it was too abstract and academic. Family health workers gave no indication of having read the memos.

#### Synergism

Synergism is a process by which individual pieces summed together produce an outcome which exceeds the sum of the individual parts. In this case, while each of the interventions we have described produced specific results, taken together these activities achieved an outcome over and above the sum of all the interventions. As one team member put it, "We have *experienced* the meaning of team. It is no longer an abstract concept." This higher order phenomenon, or "meta-learning," is the experience of the autotherapeutic process. It is demonstrated by the following outcomes:

1. The teams gained a new sense of self-control and efficacy. Many members began to sense a real team identity. One team could confront the administration as a team in support of one of its nurses. Another team could stand firmly by its rules regarding visitors to team meetings, even when faced with the risk of an administrative decision forcing them to act against their will. The awareness and ownership of their own rules, norms, feelings, successes, and failures gave the teams a greater sense of legitimacy.

2. The teams began to sense the growth of a climate in which all members could express ideas and feelings. The risk of doing this and being hurt, ridiculed, ignored, or taken for granted was now manageable. They began to experience ways to reduce the risk (and the anxiety it created) through support, feedback, trust, and openness.

### CONCLUSIONS

Our pilot work with the two teams was quickly followed by similar efforts with four other teams. This meant that by the end of the summer of 1971, six of the eight health care teams at the center had had some fifteen hours of training to help them start dealing more effectively with their own team processes.

What was the outcome? What could be accomplished in such a limited time frame? To begin with, results were somewhat uneven. Not all the teams reacted as positively as the two pilot groups. Like individuals, teams vary in their responsiveness to a training program that is new and different. If a doctor on the team was unenthusiastic or negative (which did happen), other members tended to follow his lead. And team members often found it hard to relate their training experience to their everyday work. Generally, however, the reaction to the training was positive.

But our limited time frame had other consequences. For one thing it meant that our intervention objectives of necessity had to be modest. While we observed increased clarity of role expectations, greater flexibility in decision making, and more widely shared influence and participation, the question of permanence and the relationship of these internal changes to the more ultimate measures of improved delivery of health care remain unanswered.

Actually much of the new behavior exhibited by the teams could best be described as being in the "awkward stage," which is to be expected since team members were trying to do something new and difficult for the first time. The danger here is that without some reinforcement or follow-up activities to help reduce the awkwardness, the chances of reverting to the older anxiety-driven behavior are great. If attitudes are to be changed and the new learning internalized, continuing OD support is essential. While fifteen hours is enough to initiate change and to unfreeze the teams, no team can be "OD'd" in a one-shot program and expect to be "healed" forever. OD is a process more resembling health care than a health cure.

Two things do seem clear at this point:

First, it is naïve to bring together a highly diverse group of people and to expect that, by calling them a team, they will in fact behave as a team. It is ironic indeed to realize that a football team spends 40 hours per week practicing teamwork for those two hours on Sunday afternoon when their teamwork really counts. Teams in organizations seldom spend two hours per year practicing when their ability to function as a team counts 40 hours per week!

Second, behavioral science knowledge and techniques, developed in a variety of nonmedical settings, are relevant and appear to be transferable to organizations involved in the delivery of health care.

We turn now to some broader issues and generalizations:

Whenever a team is formed to perform a task, certain predictable issues will arise which, if not effectively managed, will operate to impair the team's ability to function.

A unique connection exists between what a team does (its task) and how it goes about doing it (its internal group processes). At a very simple level, the health care analogy would be: If a team is to treat a family as an integrated unit (its task), the team itself must in many ways operate as a highly integrated family unit (its internal group processes). When a team's internal processes are inappropriate, it is likely to be no more than a collection of single entities treating subparts of single patients.

The action research model we have discussed (in this case the Kolb-Frohman model) represents a methodology and set of values that will help a team become a self-renewing or autotherapeutic organism. In some ways it demands of a team that it treat itself as a patient—periodically diagnosing its own state of health, prescribing its own medication, and subjecting itself to regular checkups to insure that the prescription is working. Although this process may require the assistance of an outsider initially, the "patient" team can learn to do many of the things itself.

The internal process issues we have discussed will occur in any group. They cannot be wished away or ignored for long without cost. Nor are they the result—as is frequently assumed—of basic personality problems. More often team members have difficulty functioning together because of ambiguous goals, unclear role expectations, dysfunctional decision making procedures, and other such process issues. These issues should be anticipated and effectively managed when they occur.

But it is not enough for the teams alone to handle their internal processes effectively. The administration supporting the teams must also be willing to experiment with flexible modes of decision making, open communication, and problem solving. One compelling reason for this is that the processes of decision making, communication, and problem solving developed at the top of an organization set norms and reinforce behavior throughout the organization. *What happens within the administration is reflected and magnified at the team and support levels.* For example, a vague decision making process by the administration seemed reflected in the MLK teams' difficulty in decision making.

The interdependencies of most modern organizations, particularly this health center, suggest that successful organization development efforts be organization-wide and managed from the top.[11] Since we know that in traditional pyramidal bureaucracies, orders are communicated from top to bottom (the first line supervisor tends to mirror the overall organization style unless he is extremely strong willed or independently wealthy), the top must set the right example. Therefore, we would like to see this health center's administration develop an image as an environmental resource available to facilitate the team delivery of health care as against, say, a collection of medical people running the place. And this is not impossible, since the administration constitutes a part of the team's life space that is capable of responding to team needs.

Undertaking such an effort would mean that rather than a traditional pyramidal organization in which the bottom supports the top, the center would become a large team, sharing needs, setting priorities, and combining resources so as to most effectively support the primary delivery system of the organization—the health teams. In this way, not only would the right hand of the center know what the left hand is doing, but the right hand would also be able to help.

## NOTES

1. Edgar Schein, *Organizational Psychology*, Englewood Cliffs, N.J.: Prentice-Hall, 1965.
2. For a broad look at the current practice of organization development see Addison-Wesley Series on OD, 1969, edited by Warren Bennis, Richard Beckhard, and Edgar Schein.
3. Conceptual support for our framework is drawn from two sources: Edgar Schein, *Organizational Psychology*, p. 70; and R.W. Revans, London, *Standards for Morale: Cause and Effect in Hospitals*, Oxford University Press, 1964, Ch. 9. Schein identifies the dual function of any group as meeting the organizational task needs and its own social needs. Revans identifies the outstanding social need of the hospital organization as the effective management of anxiety. Our assumption in the health team setting is that a certain level of "teamness" is needed to manage this anxiety, uncertainty, and frustration.
4. Harold Wise, *Fourth Annual Report of the Dr. Martin Luther King, Jr. Health Center*, 1970, p. 8.
5. For a detailed discussion of "process factors" in teams, see Edgar Schein, *Process Consultation*, Reading, Mass.: Addison-Wesley, 1969; and I. Rubin and R. Beckhard, "Factors Influencing the Effectiveness of Health Teams," *Milbank Quarterly*, July 1972, Part I. Vol. 50, pp. 317–335.
6. Edgar Schein has identified six methods by which groups come to decisions:
   - decision by lack of response (silence equals consent)
   - decision by authority (informal or formal leader makes final decision)
   - decision by minority (a few "railroad" the decision)
   - decision by majority (vote or poll taken)
   - decision by consensus (majority concur; dissenting minority is willing to go along)
   - decision by unanimous consent (all agree) E. Schein, *Process Consultation*, Reading, Mass.: Addison-Wesley, 1969, p. 58.
7. P. Lawrence and J. Lorsch, *Developing Organizations: Diagnosis and Action*, Reading, Mass.: Addison-Wesley, 1969, p. 14.
8. D. Klein, "The Defender Role," in *The Planning of Change*, W. Bennis, K. Benne, and R. Chin (eds.), New York: Holt, Rhinehart & Winston, 1969, p. 498.
9. R. Harrison, *"Role Negotiation: A Tough Minded Approach To Team Development,"* Development Research Associates, unpublished.

10. For a detailed analysis of this role and its uses in conflict management, see R. Walton, *Third Party Consultation,* Reading, Mass.: Addison-Wesley, 1969.
11. R. Beckhard, *Strategies of OD,* Reading, Mass.: Addison-Wesley, 1969, p. 9.

## Appendix

# Portrait of a Health Care Team*

*Thomas F. Plaut*

I have worked as a pediatrician on several health teams, both in New York and Kentucky. I'd like to describe the team on which I have worked for the past three years at the Dr. Martin Luther King, Jr. Health Center in the South Bronx. I will point out some strengths and weaknesses of a team and describe a few important events in the life of our team, especially the work we did with the MIT consultants.

### Background and Goals

The catchment area of the MLK Center is made up of forty-five blocks containing approximately 45,000 residents. Compared to the rest of the Bronx, this area has a high rate of venereal disease, tuberculosis, out-of-wedlock pregnancies, and families on welfare. Residents of our area accounted for half the clinic visits to Morrisania City Hospital, though they comprise only one-sixth of its population.

Forty-seven percent of the residents are Black and an equal number are Puerto Rican. The majority of these people live in four- to six-flight walkup tenements, with 17,000 living in a large housing project and a few in private homes.

The health center was founded in 1966 by Dr. Harold Wise. The center's operations are sponsored by Montefiore Hospital and funded by OEO.

Its goals were and are:

- To provide comprehensive family-centered medical care for a low income neighborhood.
- To develop training programs for nonprofessionals.
- To employ community residents.

*Based on a paper presented before the Maternal Child Health Seminar, Johns Hopkins School of Hygiene and Public Health, Baltimore, Maryland, December 1971.

- To involve community residents in policy making.
- To determine if this system is effective enough to be replicable.

Our doors were opened to patients in June 1967 in what was to become a satellite center. When the main center was opened in September 1968, MLK had between 300 and 400 employees, with eight health care teams, each responsible for a specific geographic area.

**Structure**

Team E, of which I am a member, consists of thirteen full-time people: six family health workers, two public health nurses, two internists, a pediatrician, a secretary, and a dentist. We are responsible for the health care of 1,576 families living in eleven buildings of a large city housing project. At present more than 70 percent of these families are registered for care.

| *Population* | *No. of Individuals* |
|---|---|
| Black | 1,827 |
| Latin | 2,414 |
| Other | 153 |
| Total | 4,394 |

All our patients live within three blocks of the health center.

The family health workers are community residents, each of whom joined the team after six months of training for the job. They handle housing, welfare, family, court and school problems, and provide some home health care. All six family health workers on our team are married women with from three to six children. None had worked in the health field before. Their roles and tasks are still in the process of definition.

The family health workers have been trained for a new job for which there was a theoretical need but little practical understanding. They obtain medical histories, which are often ignored; they are used as messengers by physicians and nurses. They have been unable to increase their own social and health knowledge to the degree necessary to make their work more helpful to the patient and more meaningful and satisfying to them. They have been termed "the neglected people" of the health team and health center.

A total of four nurses has filled the team's two nursing positions. Their average tenure is eighteen months, age at employment is thirty, and they had an average of seven years of nursing experience at the time they joined us. None of the nurses is a community resident. Two are Black.

The nurse is a practitioner who cares for well children and prenatal patients and provides family planning services during four half-day clinic sessions. She is the coordinator of team activities. It is her job to set priorities and see tha problems relating to families and the team itself are taken care of rather than ignored. Until November 1971, she was responsible for supervising the family health workers—making daily plans with them and reviewing their patient charts.

The jobs of the team internists and pediatrician are easy to describe. They see patients in their office eight half-days per week, care for some chronically ill patients at home, and visit hospitalized patients in rotation with their colleagues.

The following tabulation presents data on Team E members as of September 1971.

| | *Current Staff* | *Left Team* | *Avg. Tenure* | *Age When Hired* | *Job Clearly Defined* | *Minority Race (%)* | *Have Children (%)* |
|---|---|---|---|---|---|---|---|
| FHW | 6 | 3 | 26 mo. | 40 | Poor | 100 | 100 |
| PHN | 2 | 2 | 18 mo. | 30 | Fair | 50 | 50 |
| MD | 3 | 1 | 21 mo. | 33 | Good | 0 | 25 |

**Intrateam Relationships**

Some family health workers resented the nurse supervising their activities. Often they had worked at the health center longer than the nurses. They felt more knowledgeable about the problems of the community since they lived there and the nurses did not. Some felt more experienced by virtue of being older and having raised more children. Differences in background and race also led to misunderstanding and discord. Hostility was at times real and at other times imagined.

In order to give the family health workers more responsibility and to provide them with an opportunity for growth, they were removed from the supervision of the public health nurses in November 1971. They may still call on the nurses and physicians freely for help; but they answer only to the medical care evaluation committee and the team as a whole for their performance.

When the team was formed three years ago, the two nurses resisted the efforts of the pediatrician to help in the supervision of the family health workers. Although they wanted to develop their own competence as practitioners before concerning themselves too much with this aspect of the job, at the same time they wanted the supervisory role to be open to them when they became ready for it.

The pediatrician was responsible for teaching the nurses well child care and provided consultation when requested. This worked out well. However, it took six months before the nurses and pediatrician could work together on team matters (as distinguished from pediatric matters) without friction. At that time, they began planning weekly team meetings together and working out plans for family care.

While the internists on the team have always been competent and conscientious in caring for their patients, they never took any intiative in working to improve the function of the team until after MIT consultants were brought into the center in February 1971 (which I will discuss later). Since that time an understanding of team membership has developed on their part and they have begun to hold informal teaching sessions for family health workers, which are well received.

The team meets as a body once a week for one and a half hours to discuss families with difficult problems or problems from which we can learn. We also exchange information of common interest. Since the MIT intervention I have been meeting weekly with the nurses. These meetings deal with common pediatric problems and enable the nurses to take over more clinical duties. I also meet weekly with the family health workers to discuss specific patients as well as general problems affecting patients.

By spending more time with the family health workers and nurses, the physicians are now demonstrating their respect for them. This demonstration of respect has been followed by a decrease in friction between physicians and other team members.

An example of genuine teamwork occurred in August 1971. At that time, the health center found that a new census was urgently needed for planning and billing purposes. The physicians decided to share this tedious but necessary job with their teammates. Every member of Team E participated in the census—several on evenings and weekends. This happened in no other team.

### Extrateam Relationships

Many outside demands are made on team members. The physicians and nurses have conflicting loyalties. The nurse, for instance, is involved with the nursing group, the pediatric nurse practitioner program, the obstetric program, covering other nurses, and outside organizations. Physicians are involved with weekly pediatric or internal medicine meetings, emergency room coverage, covering other physicians, hospitalized patients, the intern-residency program, and health center committees. The family health workers, in contrast, generally owe their allegiance to and get their primary support from the team.

### Important Events in the Life of Team E

| | |
|---|---|
| September 1968: | Formation<br>Continuous staff changes |
| December 1968: | Successfully confronted the health center administration: limited visitors to team meetings. |
| February 1971: | MIT consultation: Improved communication, growing awareness that our satisfaction is important in contributing to teamwork. |

| | |
|---|---|
| April 1971: | Fired psychiatric consultant. |
| July 1971: | Health center administration changed. |
| August 1971: | Unit management system begins: includes team's involvement in hiring. |
| November 1971: | Family health workers removed from supervision by nurses. |

There has recently been a change in the way team members relate to the administration. Before August 1971, they related to and brought problems to the health center administration through their respective peer groups: nurses, pediatricians, internists, family health workers. There was no system of team advocacy. The team often had no say and was merely informed of a change in its life—e.g., you will get two interns February 1; Professor A will visit your team conference as an observer; Dr. B will become your second internist; you will care for the following new families, etc. Starting in August of 1971, the team became responsible for hiring its own staff, approving leaves of absence and controlling intake of new registrants. Our team had asserted some autonomy previously by restricting visitors and firing a psychiatrist. In each case, facing a common "enemy" brought a feeling of unity and togetherness.

**The MIT Intervention**

I have already referred to the MIT consultation. Now I'd like to describe their goals, methods, materials and effect on the team. Professor Irwin Rubin and his student Ron Fry came to us under the auspices of the Carnegie Foundation, which is interested in the operation of health care teams. We first met them at a general medical staff meeting in January 1971, at which they described the consultation process. They stated that their goal was to help the team help itself function more effectively. They asked that the teams interested in working with them list the pros and cons of consultation as they saw them. From a group of six interested teams, the MIT people chose two, mainly on the basis of understanding of the consultation process and the unanimity of the decision.

Rubin and Beckhard have described their method as consisting of four parts: data collection, summary and feedback, action planning, and evaluation. This is exactly how Rubin and Fry worked with Team E. Each team member was interviewed for an hour and a half on such process related factors as team goals, priority setting, role definition, decision making, support and feedback among team members, and whether the team member experienced a sense of accomplishment in his work. These data were summarized and fed back to the team at its first meeting with the consultants.

Team members were surprised to see that they were not alone in their judgments and feelings about the team. Rubin and Fry discussed the material with us and suggested that we take as our initial task the improvement of our weekly team meeting, since these meetings involved all team members and we all agreed they needed improving. To this end, we took the following actions: used a planning committee to develop an agenda for the meetings, rotated chairmanship among all team members, and started on time. A written evaluation occupied the last ten minutes of each meeting. The comments were later used by the planning committee in preparing for the next meeting.

The same format of data collection, feedback, planning and evaluation was used in small groups also. The three physicians met and each wrote a recommendation for each of the other two to follow at the next meeting. The recommendations for one physician were:

1. Do not repeat yourself until others have responded. You may have been understood perfectly the first time.
2. Be more concise.
3. Do not be the first one to always fill quiet spaces.
4. Improve listening skills.

Adherence to these recommendations was discussed by the physicians at the end of the next meeting and the improvement in behavior was supported Our consultants also supplied us with tracts discussing feedback, chairing a meeting, and role negotiation.

We met with our consultants for a total of sixteen hours over a two-month period. In all our dealings with them they emphasized the importance of openness and support among team members. I believe they were successful in what they tried to do. Last week, eight months after the intervention, I polled my teammates. In the words of one family health worker: "I feel more important. The importance of everyone's job has been explained, and I am more efficient. As for other team members, they are more considerate, more willing to give. The new teaching program is a good example of this."

**Effectiveness of the Team**

What gives a team strength? A feeling of accomplishment which brings satisfaction; a feeling of working together for a common goal. The feeling of accomplishment can come only if one has a clear-cut goal which is attainable in a reasonable period of time. Crash immunization programs are a beautiful example of this: everybody feels great when the measurable accomplishments are read off at the end of a single day.

The members of Team E at the Dr. Martin Luther King, Jr. Health Center have an unending job. The goal set out for us to bring to an optimal state of health all 6,200 individuals living in our area can never be attained with our resources. We haven't even agreed upon the components of the goal. In short, although we are the best team at the best health center in the country, there is plenty of room for improvement.

**Growth Stages Required for Teamwork at MLK**

Each individual must go through the following stages before he can function as part of a team. The time spent at each stage varies with the personality, previous experience, competence, job category, stage of fellow workers, and other responsibilities. Advancement may occur in several areas at the same time.

1. *Groping.* Everyone starts here. No one knows his or her role or tasks. Evidenced by purposeless movement or by inaction.
2. *Orientation to tasks and roles.* Easy for physician–because trained for majority of his tasks. Hard for nurse because of quadruple role and previous training in only one area. Impossible for most family health workers until the rest of the team gets itself together to support her.
3. *Development of individual competence.* Once this has been achieved, a helping role becomes possible.
4. *Reorientation.* Necessary for MD with regard to relationships to teammates and also to new tasks–for example, community orientation.
5. *Setting priorities.* When several people are oriented and competent they can join together to set priorities and work together, bringing their teammates along.

## About Chapter Three

*Team improvement efforts, to be successful, not only need reinforcing at the team level but also require the support of the organization's overall administrative structure. If management has reason to suspect that the administrative structure does not support lower levels in the organization, how does it go about determining what exactly needs to be changed? Do a group of experts, working in splendid isolation, formulate answers to what ails the organization–based on good management principles and practices, plain common sense, or what another organization has found successful?*

*If this is the approach used in planning change–and it often is–the effort is unlikely to be rewarding. For no matter how bright or how capable these planners may be, if they have not collected the basic facts, the basic data they need, from the organization itself, their solutions are not likely to work. Yet it is a strange fact of life that managers will often seek solutions anywhere except within their own organizations.*

*However, if we assume that our managers are not burdened with this reluctance, that they want the facts wherever they are, the question then is: What data do they need? What in the organization should they be examining?*

*In Chapter Three, Richard Beckhard looks at six key categories against which organizational effectiveness can be measured. These include such basics as the organization's structure as it relates to the organization's work, communication and information flow, and decision making. When data relating to these various categories are analyzed, management should be in an excellent position to initiate a successful planned change effort.*

*Using the MLK Center as an example, Beckhard describes how an organization can restructure itself to more effectively achieve its objectives. In the process, he highlights some basic principles of organization that should be helpful to managers and administrators in many fields.*

Chapter Three

# Organizational Implications of Team Building: The Larger Picture

*Richard Beckhard*

The critical and growing problem of providing comprehensive health care to an expanding patient population is dramatized in poor communities, where the shortage of trained medical personnel is acute and the needs of families for a variety of health and social services escalate daily. Public and private agencies are accelerating their efforts to deal with this problem.

Many of these efforts involve the creation of interdisciplinary health care teams. The Department of Health, Education, and Welfare is today actively recruiting such teams for use throughout the country. Hospitals are experimenting with team delivery of ambulatory care. And community health centers are using interdisciplinary teams, with the family as the patient unit.

Administrators of such centers face many new and complex issues in trying to manage them. There are issues around the organization of the health team, the structure of the total organization, educational policy and practices, staff motivation, and community relations—to name but a few.

Where can the administrators look for help in trying to achieve their difficult goals? The answer, I believe, lies in a body of experience, mostly in non-medical organizations, where the application of behavioral science-based knowledge has significantly improved organizational effectiveness. I believe that some of this knowledge and experience can be of considerable assistance in the administration of team delivered, community-based comprehensive health care.

In this chapter I will look at a number of organizational issues that arose at the Dr. Martin Luther King, Jr. Health Center and relate them to the methods used in other settings to analyze and improve an organization's effectiveness.[1] Specifically, I will examine the kinds of organization problems that exist in a community-based health center. Then I will identify several ways of looking at organizational functioning and apply these methods to the organization problems I have identified. Finally, I will discuss some implications for the curricula of medical and professional schools concerned with the education and training of health workers for the practice of social medicine.

## ORGANIZATIONAL ISSUES

"Let me describe our major problems as I see them." The director of the Dr. Martin Luther King, Jr. Health Center is talking.

> Health care is delivered to the families in the community through health teams composed of physicians, nurses and community-based and center-trained family health workers. We are having a lot of difficulties in the operation of the health teams.
>
> We have problems with the role of the public health nurse on the teams. She is assigned as the coordinator and leader of the health team but this is a very strange role for her.
>
> We have a lot of communication difficulties between the community oriented family health workers and the professionally trained physicians and nurses.
>
> We are having a number of problems with supervision, particularly first-line supervisors who are mostly community residents whom we have trained.
>
> We're having a lot of difficulty around information flow and record keeping. Patient records are often incomplete and in the wrong place at the wrong time. A number of referrals get lost between departments and between the center and the hospital.
>
> Another problem for me is that the top team doesn't function very much as a team. Each functional department head, such as pediatrics or obstetrics, has his functional counterparts on the delivery team reporting to him and tends, naturally, to be more concerned with his own functional area than with the overall management of the center. This makes it difficult to get best decisions for the whole organization.
>
> We're pretty sure that we're not properly organized structurally to manage this operation, but we don't know exactly how we should change our organization.

### Cause of the Problems

If we are to adequately define the problems arising from these multiple issues outlined by the center's director, we first need to look at the environmental situation.

There are two environments or "systems" interacting: the *patient system* with its problems, desires, and needs; and the *health care delivery system*, which is composed of a variety of subsystems, such as medical practitioners, community development workers, educators, and administrators.

If we analyze these two systems as they were operating in MLK, the following facts emerge:

The patient system is highly complex. The patient families are composed of individuals with a variety of physical, emotional, and social problems.

They present a varied set of needs for service—treatment of disease, maintenance of health, improvement of living conditions, education in health and citizenship, and assistance in bringing about change in their community.

They also have a variety of expectations concerning the health center staff—treatment of illness; advice on citizen rights; getting public agencies to take some action on community problems; leadership in dealing with social problems such as drug abuse or rat infestation; getting information on health matters such as prenatal care and birth control.

The health care delivery system (the primary care health team plus a backup of medical and social specialties) is composed of a variety of specialists who are trained to deal with one or at most a few of the types of needs and expectations of the patient system. But the health problems of the patient system tend to be interdependent and complex. For example, lack of adequate heat due to an absentee landlord causes the family to have more sickness such as colds and flu. If such complex problems are to be adequately dealt with, the center must have capabilities in many areas:

1. Evaluating health problems.
2. Diagnosing disease causes.
3. Treatment of medical problems.
4. Diagnosing and evaluating social and economic problems.
5. Treating social problems by legal or social action.
6. Maintaining a family's condition once it is improved.

The total services needed cannot be effectively delivered by assigning parts of the problem to specialists on the delivery team trained to treat those parts. Rather, what is required is an integrated effort by a number of different health workers to treat the complex problems of the patient family. And because of this, it is necessary for all health workers on a team:

1. To understand the total complex of health problems of their patient families.
2. To understand the patients' needs, attitudes, expectations, and values.
3. To be able to jointly assess what resources (members of the health team and backup specialists) can best be deployed for diagnosis, treatment, health maintenance, and education of the patient families.

### Issues for the Leaders

Given the variety of needs and expectations of patient families; the various educational, technical, and social backgrounds of the medical and social health workers; the necessity to have integrated team diagnoses and treatment of the interrelated medical and social problems in patient families, the organization's leadership is faced with a series of questions, each starting with, "how can we:

1. Help the primary care teams integrate their diagnosis and treatment of their patient populations?
2. Provide an organization structure that reflects the work requirements?
3. Deal with the human problems arising from a situation where physicians, nurses and family health workers have to collaboratively perform a variety of tasks, many of them never before performed by these people?
4. Locate authority and develop competence so that decisions are made by those who possess the best information and are closest to the problem?
5. Build an information system and communication network that assures that all health workers have the best available information?
6. Build "linkages" between the practitioners (primary care teams) and the support system (all others)?
7. Develop education and training programs that assure
   a. Adequate dissemination of clinical content to a variety of health workers.
   b. Dissemination of content about the social conditions of patient families and the community culture to medical practitioners.
   c. Develop training in group membership skills for a variety of health workers.
   d. Provide adequate training in leadership and supervision for health team leaders, medical administrators, and medical practitioners.
8. Maintain a patient oriented system in a situation where there are strong forces to mass produce the care?
9. Keep a staff with a variety of different backgrounds and values motivated and working together?"

Given this set of organization problems, the administrator is in need of some consistent framework within which he can approach the various issues. It is here that the methods of organization analysis and planning used in other settings are most useful.

## ORGANIZATION EFFECTIVENESS

There are several categories against which organization effectiveness can be measured:

1. The effectiveness of work teams.
2. Organization structure and its relationship to the work.
3. The types of tasks and the roles needed to perform them.
   a. Job descriptions and their use.
   b. Job enrichment and modification.
4. Decision making.
5. Communications and information flow.
6. Education and development strategy.

We will now examine each of these six categories in some detail.

**Team Effectiveness**

As we have already seen, a major leadership question is "How to help primary care teams integrate their diagnosis and treatment of the total health problems of their patient population?" But first, before examining team effectiveness as a category, some definitions.

A *team* is a group with a specific task or tasks, the accomplishment of which requires the interdependent and collaborative efforts of its members. To illustrate, a group of physicians who share an office, but each of whom has his own patients, would not fit this definition of a team. But a surgical team working in an operating room would.

*Effectiveness* implies that the greatest part of the group's energy is focused on accomplishing its tasks. Minimum energy is required for "maintaining" the group—its morale, its member satisfaction, and its work processes. Here again, most surgical teams are excellent examples of team effectiveness.

In the community ambulatory setting, however, a number of conditions tend to work against high effectiveness. Table 3–1 lists a few of these factors and compares them with the surgical team environment.

As Table 3–1 indicates, the situation in which the community health team functions tends to be ambiguous. People are much less clear about what is expected of them. Competition for leadership is more likely to occur. Because of different priorities, decisions are harder to make and frequently are not made. Communication is likely to be closed because people are not sure of the consequences of being open. In the health teams I observed in the center, all these behaviors occurred.

To deal with such a set of conditions it is imperative that the team spend some time, preferably early in its life, explicitly examining how it will work. It needs to come to grips with such issues as:

1. Which members will perform which work?
2. How will this be decided?
3. What problems of patient identification, diagnosis, treatment, health maintenance, and patient education need to be dealt with by the team working as a group?
4. What are the role expectations of each member for the others? For example, what does the physician expect of the public health nurse? How does this fit her expectations?
5. What information is needed from one member by another? For example, what does the pediatrician, who sees the patient in his office, need to know from the family health worker, who visits the family at home, about the life style, values, and living conditions of the patient's family?
6. What personal and professional development needs does each member have? How can the team help meet these needs?

**Table 3–1. Comparison of Surgical Team to Health Care Team**

| *Condition* | *Surgical Team* | *Community Primary Care Team* |
|---|---|---|
| Purpose | Specific: to operate and heal | General: comprehensive care |
| Task | Very clear | Somewhat unclear: probably many tasks |
| Who does what? | Roles and functions very clear | Roles ambiguous: several members may perform same functions for different patients |
| Where work is performed | In one location | In a number of locations |
| Decision making | Clear hierarchy: surgeon, first assistant, scrub nurse | Unclear: group of colleagues with different information and skills; group decisions sometimes required |
| Communication | One-way command system | May be discussive and problem solving |
| Goal priorities | Same for all members | May vary among members (medical treatment vs. social action vs. education) |

To work effectively on these problems of team development probably requires assistance from someone skilled in helping a team look at such issues. He or she may be an outside organization development consultant, an education specialist within the organization, or a member of the institution's management trained in these skills.

In any case, community health care centers should, I believe, develop a capability for helping delivery teams to consciously work on improving their own internal effectiveness through examining their own processes, practices, and relationships.

**Organization Structure and Its Relationship to Work**

The question, "What is the most appropriate structure around which to organize the task?" is a universal organizational issue. It is particularly important in settings such as community ambulatory care where the work is so varied and relies on so many different technical backgrounds.

In such delivery systems, the practitioners (the deliverers of health care) tend to be located at the bottom of the organizational totem pole. Family health workers, public health nurses, physicians—these are the people who actually deliver the care; everybody else in the organization is there to support their efforts. Yet the organization chart often shows a very different picture. For example, Figure 3–1 shows a traditional hospital oriented reporting system, which is the one originally used in the MLK Center.

Each specialist (pediatrician, internist, nurse) reported directly to his/her functional counterpart. Family health workers who had no counterpart reported to the public health nurse. A structure such as this does not support the teams; rather it maintains the separation of team members by having them report up functional lines.

If we redraw the chart from the point of view of the services to be delivered (as the King Center did) the result can be seen in Figure 3–2. In this chart all members of a health team report to a unit manager who is the administrative boss. His job is to facilitate the team delivery of health care. The chiefs of service are supports—technical and educational resources available to guide, counsel, and plan with all team members.

These two charts represent two major types of structure: *functional*—based on technology (medical specialties); and *product-service*—based on "market" (patient needs and demands). However, the nature of the requirements for service in this setting, including preventive care, treatment care, and improvement of social conditions, probably means that a third organization structure—a matrix design—is required. A matrix type of structure is used in complex organizations when the interdependencies around work are such that no simple reporting structure such as the pyramid type of organization will do.

Let me describe a matrix structure. We find a series of *operating*

**Figure 3–1.** Traditional Organization Chart

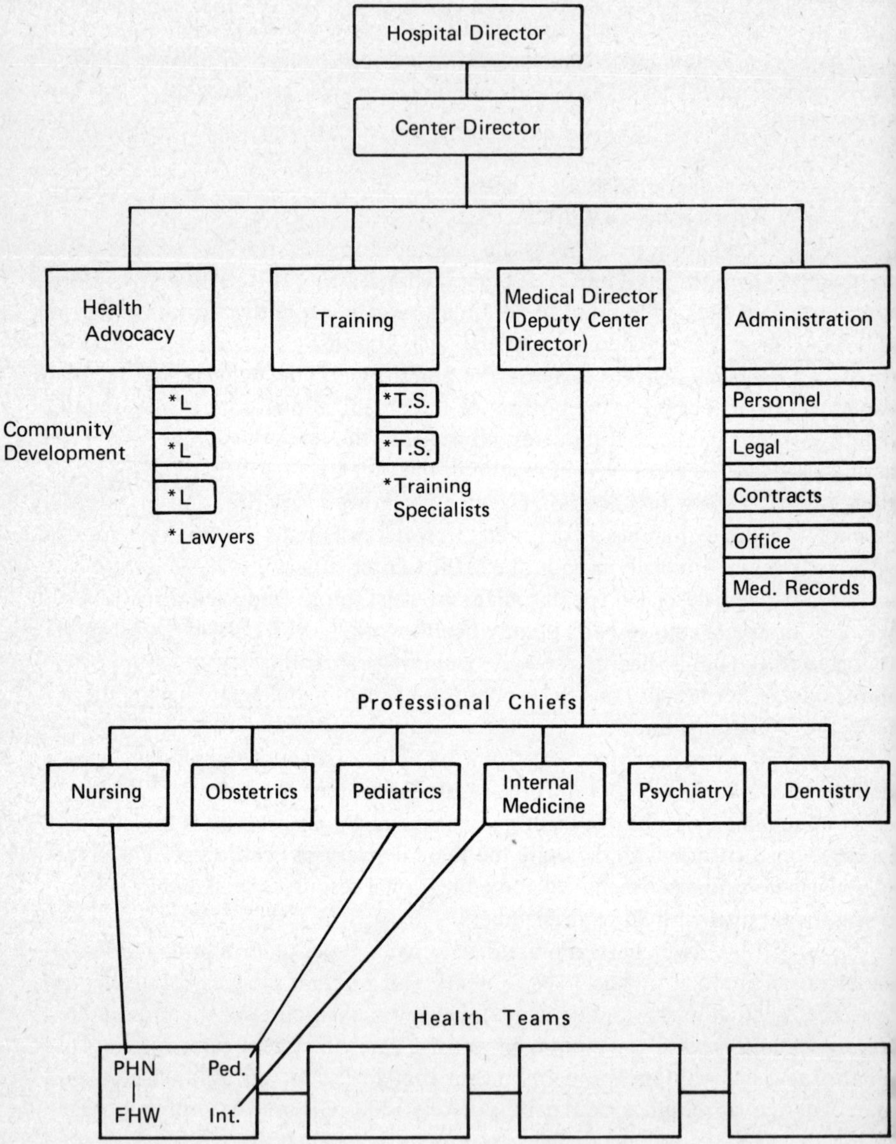

**Figure 3–2.** Organization Chart Based on Product and Service

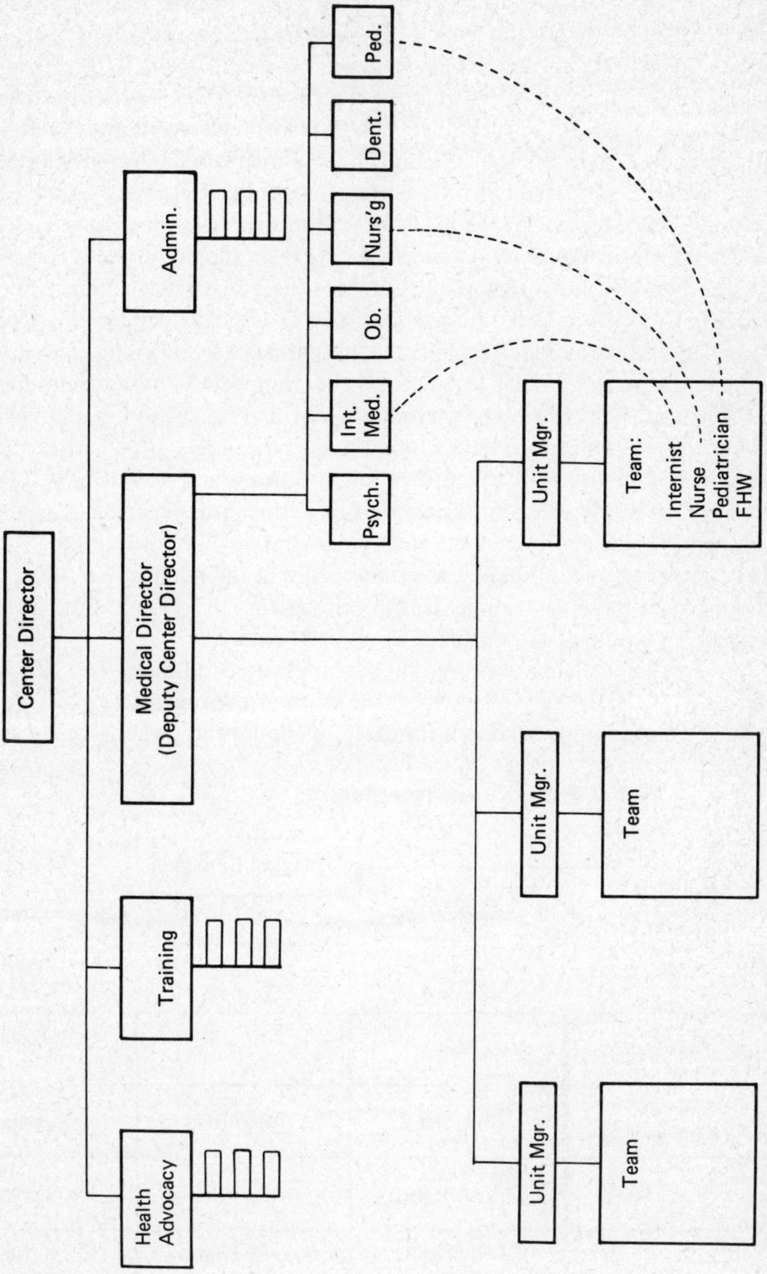

*units,* such as health teams; and a set of *capabilities,* such as internal medicine, psychiatry, dentistry, etc. The operating units and the capabilities must interact regularly in order to get the work done. A variety of combinations of people will need to collaborate around specific tasks.

Figure 3–3 shows a matrix chart for the MLK Center. Here we see a series of operating units (in this case health teams) and a series of capabilities, such as medical specialties, both reporting to a medical director. The operating units might be compared to profit centers in an industrial organization. Each is responsible for "a piece of the business." The capabilities, such as obstetrics, psychiatry, and community organization, are technology resources. The management problem for the director is to combine these operating centers and capabilities in ways which will optimize the delivery of health services.

For example, the public health nurse on the team not only reports to the unit manager but she also needs to be "supported" by the chief nurse regarding nursing practice and the training of other nurses and family health workers. She also needs to have a direct line to the chiefs of pediatrics and internal medicine relative to the identification, diagnosis, and treatment of disease. In addition, she needs access to the training and education department around development needs, and to medical and administrative directors relative to supervisory and personnel problems, as well as issues in the relationship of her team to other parts of the organization. This multireporting situation is quite different from the typical medical organization reporting lines.

To make matters even more complicated, all these reporting lines refer only to the delivery of services—the work of the organization. In addition, a separate reporting line is needed for career planning and personal development.

**Figure 3–3.** Matrix Structure

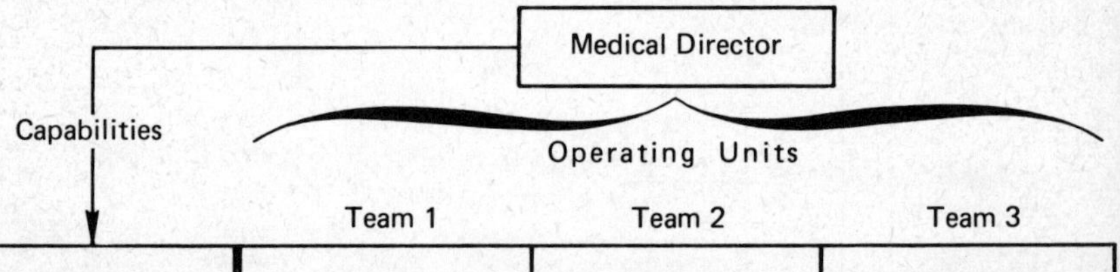


| | Team 1 | Team 2 | Team 3 |
|---|---|---|---|
| Nursing | PHN | PHN | PHN |
| Internal Medicine | Internist | Internist | Internist |
| Pediatrics | Pediatrician | Pediatrician | Pediatrician |
| | Family Health Worker | Family Health Worker | Family Health Worker |

For this purpose, a functional hierarchy is usually appropriate. Thus our nurse probably reports to the chief nurse for her own career planning and personal development. The chief nurse, in turn, needs to coordinate with the medical director in regard to career opportunities, career paths, and career ladders for the nurse who might want to move out of her present role into administrative or physician's assistant roles.

One more complication. There probably needs to be a separate organization structure for organization planning and development. The capabilities and relationships needed to operate the day-to-day services are not the same as those required for planning the future of the organization. Many nonmedical organizations have a separate organization chart for future planning. I suspect administrators of health centers would be wise to also consider this.

To summarize, organizations are in fact multistructured. Realistic managements recognize this and explicitly design their structural charts to reflect this fact. It is my belief that health centers in the future are also likely to adopt multiple organization structures.

However, it is important to recognize that working in such a structure is much more demanding than in the traditional structure. Authority is less clearly defined, decision making is more complex, the situation is more ambiguous—all of which tend to produce tension and anxiety among the members of the organization. In an attempt to deal with this anxiety, some organizations move to tighten up the structure and return to clear lines of authority, with decision making recentralized at the top. But this is not the answer. What has to be realized is that the situation *is* ambiguous and anxiety producing—and necessarily so. Rather than attempting to reduce the anxiety by reverting to old organizational models that are not effective it is much more productive to use the energy in developing specific structures to fit the work to be done, focusing on patient needs and requirements. Reporting should be based more on information needs than on authority or power.

A guiding rule for administrators should be: "Form follows function."

### Tasks and Roles

Our third category against which to measure organization effectiveness is the degree of understanding of tasks and roles by the persons performing the work. These people need to understand what their jobs are, both in terms of their own wishes and in terms of the expectations of the relevant people around them.

In studies of organizations, this phenomenon is called a "role set"—that is, the person in a role, such as nurse or pediatrician, finds himself in the middle of a cluster of expectations about how he should perform in that role. His boss, subordinates, and relevant colleagues all have expectations concerning him, which may or may not dovetail with each other and with his own values and desires. Figure 3–4 shows the role set of a public health nurse who is a team coordinator in a community health center.

When one examines the many expectations she is faced with, it is obvious that she cannot meet all of them at any one time. This often produces a condition of role conflict.

**Figure 3–4.** Role Set of Public Health Nurse

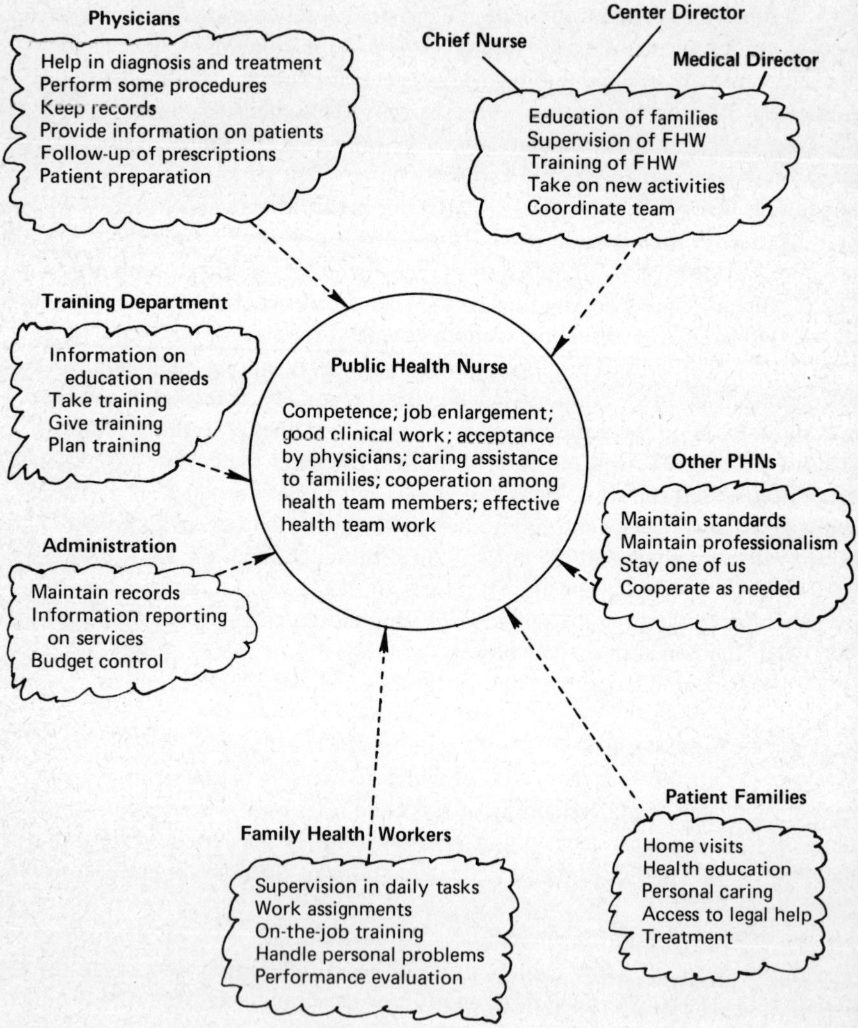

Role conflict is minimized in most hospital settings because the role titles (internist, obstetrician, surgical nurse) define the types of tasks the incumbent will perform as well as the relationships he will have with other roles. But in the community setting, where the roles are considerably less clearly defined, the conflict is greater.

Look at Figure 3–4 again. How can the nurse determine priorities for spending her time? How much of her energy should be devoted to: Delivering services to patients? Learning new skills and procedures? Visiting patient families? Supervising the work of family health workers? Educating and training other workers? Learning about supervision and management?

Nor can decisions about how she will use her time and energy be made by the nurse alone, or by her supervisor, since such decisions affect and are affected by at least ten other people. Because of the many pulls and tugs this situation creates, people often retreat to doing those things they already know how to do and feel comfortable doing. If this is the case with our nurse, she will give priority to the old aspects of her job for which she has had previous training and practice, while ignoring unfamiliar areas, even though the latter might be most needed for patients or would free up physicians to do things for which they alone have the capability.

The problem can be somewhat lessened if specific criteria are developed to help make these choices. Criteria that might be considered in this case are shown in Table 3–2.

By working with these or other criteria the nurse should be able to develop a priority system for the use of her own time. Then, in collaboration with some of her most relevant colleagues, she is in a position to make the best possible decisions. In any case, it is essential that specific means of choosing are developed.

**Table 3–2. Criteria Used to Set Priorities**

| | | | |
|---|---|---|---|
| Direct service to patients | Low | ______________ | High |
| Short/long term effects | Short | ______________ | Long |
| Immediate effects on other workers | Few | ______________ | Many |
| If neglected now, what's the cost? | Low | ______________ | High |
| How important is it to me? | Not very | ______________ | Very |

**Job Descriptions:** In most organizations, management seeks to clarify roles by developing job descriptions. These attempt to define the tasks, responsibilities, and authority of someone doing a particular piece of work. Usual assumptions behind this practice are: (1) a job can be defined with sufficient specificity for any person to do it in pretty much the same manner; (2) a variety of people can "fit into a job description"; (3) the work is similar enough in a variety of different situations to produce a universal description.

But in recent years, in many nonmedical organizations where the work has become more complex and the people more insistent that they be treated as individuals, traditional job descriptions, usually developed by a personnel department or a functional department head, have proved to be nonfunctional and frequently dysfunctional to both work and morale. Managers have found it necessary to develop a specific man-job description for each situation. To take one example, the specifics of the job description for the astronauts in Apollo 16 differed from those in Apollo 18, based on a different though similar mission, different specific tasks, and different "performers" in the same role.

A more realistic assumption in describing jobs is "a job is a man in action." For example, imagine two foremen in an industrial organization assigned to the same job in two work areas.

*Foreman A* *Foreman B*

While there are a number of tasks which both of these men must perform, there is latitude in the way in which the tasks are performed, the personal styles of *A* and *B*, and the setting in which the work is performed. So, more realistically, *A*'s job looks like

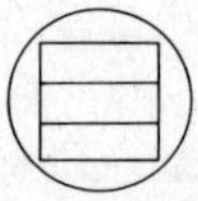

while *B*'s job looks like

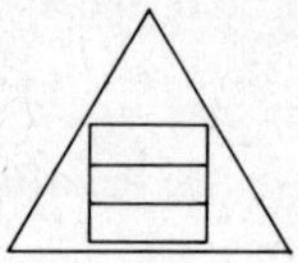

The most realistic job description would be one that accurately described *A* or *B* doing the job.

To apply this to our community health center we might look, for example, at the role of the family health worker and some of the factors that affect how each individual performs the job.

The family health worker is a community resident who has been selected to be a member of a health team. She (or he) has received six months of training in nursing, social work, and community development. She then joins a health team composed of two public health nurses, a pediatrician, an internist, and five other family health workers, which services some 1,500 patient families in a multiblock area.

To define her job the following must be considered:

1. Each health team serves a different patient population.
2. The priorities of demands for service vary as a result of social, economic, ethnic, and other characteristics.
3. Each health team has a unique internal operating mode. In Team A the family health worker may spend most of her time making home visits, and taking down basic information on health conditions. In Team B her work may include taking a leadership role in helping to correct substandard housing conditions, aggressive patient recruitment, and teaching the medical staff about the conditions of the patient families.

No single job description could possibly reflect these differences.

What has been found to be more appropriate in other settings and, I suspect, has application in this setting, is to develop a "living description."

In this case the family health worker would write down her picture of the job as she performs it. Her description is then checked with her supervisor and relevant colleagues (such as other team members and service heads). The resulting description reflects the understanding of the person in the job and the relevant people around her about what work she is to do.

Such a procedure also provides a practical benchmark for planning performance improvement and for performance evaluation.

**Job Modification and Enrichment**: Another dimension to consider in the tasks and roles category is job enrichment and job modification. If we look at the work requirements and compare them with what is actually being done by whom, we often find that the best use is not being made of a particular capability. For example, applying this yardstick to the tasks and capabilities of the chiefs of service in the MLK Center produced some major changes in job emphasis and activities. A few examples follow.

Prior to the organizational examination, the heads of pediatrics, internal medicine, nursing, etc., were (1) *responsible* for the work of their functional counterparts; (2) *responsible* for discipline of their functional counterparts; (3) *responsible* for the education of their functional counterparts; and (4) *responsible* for the application of their specialty to patient service.

After a review by the incumbent heads of service as to how best to use their talents in terms of the total mission of the center, the priorities changed. A more current description of their responsibilities includes:

1. Leadership in reviewing and disseminating information about the commonly encountered disease problems in the patient population. An example would be to develop information on treating diabetic patients at the center as well

as guidelines to help teams decide who should be trained to do what about this particular health problem.
2. Clinical education for a variety of health workers with different backgrounds, which means both teaching and helping others to teach.
3. Setting quality standards and guidelines.
4. Consultation on problems in their specialty.

You will note that two important items in the earlier description—responsibility for discipline of counterparts (2) and responsibility for the application of their specialty to the patient population (4)—and part of a third—the responsibility for the education of their functional counterparts (3)—were transferred to the teams themselves and to team management.

To summarize about tasks and roles: people need to understand what is expected of them; in new fields and turbulent settings, a variety of expectations exist, which in the community health care setting produces competition for the time of the health worker. Therefore criteria need to be developed to choose among the competitors; man-in-job descriptions provide this kind of information. Finally, by looking at *work,* jobs can be enlarged and enriched and made more relevant to patient requirements.

**Decision Making**

Most nonmedical organizations have traditionally located decisions at the level of the hierarchy that most closely corresponds to the degree of risk involved. For example, \$5,000 decisions are made at one level, \$10,000 at the next level, and so forth. But as customer demands (as well as the organization required to meet them) have grown in complexity, this basis for decision making has proven to be no longer adequate. Neither is it in community medical practice, I suspect.

Today, in complex organizations, there is a strong trend toward having decisions made (a) as close to the problem as possible and (b) by those who have the relevant information, regardless of their role or location in the organizational hierarchy. In a health delivery system, a first question might relate to the location of information, particularly about patients' needs.

In the community setting, information is located in several places—some in the patient, some in the family health worker, some in the nurse, some in the physician. Figure 3–5 illustrates this pattern. Since in this case the information all comes together in the primary care health team, it makes sense for decisions of the following kinds to be located there.

1. Evaluation of patient health.
2. Diagnosis of health problems.
3. Treatment of health problems.
4. Strategies for recruiting patients.

**Figure 3–5.** Information About Patient Needs

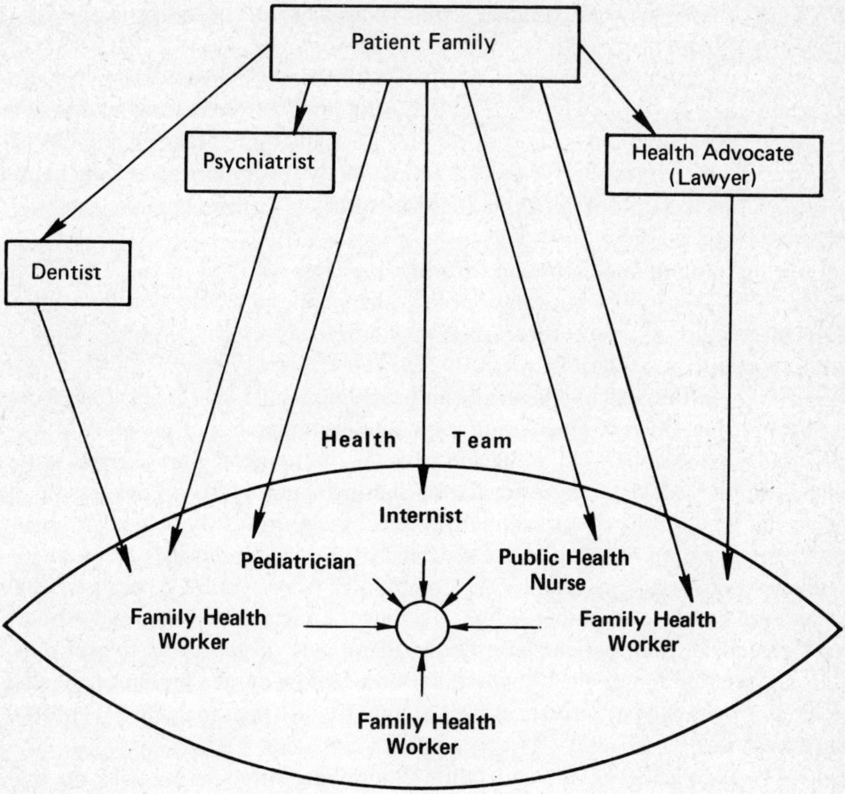


5. Strategies for educating patients.
6. Application of clinical knowledge such as disease treatment to a specific patient population.
7. Work plans and scheduling of team members.
8. Group conferences for sharing information and problems.
9. Administrative and housekeeping matters.

But for management to simply reassign such decision making to the health teams may not work. At the MLK Center, where health team members had had little or no experience in handling such administrative matters, specialized training in both decision making and how to process information was required before the team could effectively implement decisions. Some structural changes were also needed to handle the administrative decisions—for example, the role of unit manager was created. The incumbent in this role, who reports to the medical director, is responsible for scheduling team members' work and providing a linkage to the rest of the organization. Decisions around the delivery of health care have also been assigned to the teams or to subgroups or task forces made up of team members.

To summarize, organization effectiveness is increased when: (1) decisions are made by those who have the requisite information (example, decisions about education, patient relationships, etc. are made by the teams); and (2) administrators recognize that "people are most likely to support what they help to create." "Ownership" of decisions goes far toward effective implementation.

**Communications and Information Flow**

The flow of information, the quality of communication in terms of its openness, and the type of information transmitted within an organization are important factors against which to measure effectiveness.

In the case of a health team providing family-centered care in a community setting, it is extremely important that each member of the team know what all other members are doing and why they're doing it. This requires much more communication, more information sharing, and a degree of openness and trust that may not be so critical in other settings. Although typical health teams today are made up of a number of specialists (physicians, nurses, community workers), the services needed by the community often require generalists. Physicians need to know a number of things about the social conditions and ethnic backgrounds of their patients in order to adequately diagnose and treat. Community oriented family health workers need to know quite a bit about the diagnosis and treatment of disease, as well as how to deal with social problems in the neighborhood.

To achieve these ends, time should be allotted for working on communication problems and information flow, since we know that teams do benefit from analyzing their communication processes. The analysis might include the kinds of information that need to be shared, the direction of information (who needs to know what), and the identification of linkages between parts of the organization, such as team to team, team to medical department heads, or team to administrative services.

On the basis of this kind of analysis, various procedures such as meetings, memoranda, reporting forms can be devised that will facilitate the work. For example, a communication analysis at the MLK Center showed that middle management department heads such as medical records, pharmacy, etc. felt quite removed from the top management group. Information on plans, priorities, treatment practices was not shared. Simultaneously, the middle managers were withholding information from the central group.

From this finding it was a relatively easy step to set up monthly joint meetings, to initiate a feedback system that could operate between meetings to assure the flow of necessary information, and to create a task group among several levels to continually monitor the communications.

Clearly there is a great need today in complex health delivery institutions to develop comprehensive information systems that will optimize the flow of information, both technical and administrative. While I do not propose at this point to go into detail about information systems, I do want to call the reader's attention to the availability of a body of knowledge on the subject, which could well be applied more effectively than it is at present in community and social medicine management.

**Education and Development Strategy**

An important variable in any organization is how it manages the development of its staff. Good management must concern itself both with organizing the day-to-day work and organizing to manage the training and development of people for advancement and enrichment.

In the community comprehensive-care setting, many new issues focusing on education and development need to be considered. Two are:

1. What clinical content needs to be taught to what staff roles? For example, who—physicians, nurses, family health workers—needs to know and be able to do what about the diagnosis and treatment of diabetes in this community?
2. What content should be taught in the team setting and what content should be taught in professional peer groups?

In many medical settings senior doctors teach junior doctors and senior nurses teach junior nurses. The student is in a "classroom" of his peers. In the community setting, however, there are a number of important reasons for teaching both medical *and* management content to the practicing team. First, the application of the content to the specific patient problems can be effectively carried out only by team members; second, for team development purposes this type of activity provides an ideal situation for collaborative effort among a number of members.

To again draw an analogy from the space program, all astronauts receive similar basic training in a variety of technical work, problem solving, etc. However, when a particular team is assigned a specific mission, such as Apollo 16, the training for that mission is given to the total team in the team setting. The team is composed of the astronauts who will fly, the backup team who may fly the mission, and the capsule communicators—fellow astronauts who are "flying the mission" from the ground. Success depends on these people "being in each other's heads"—each knowing how the others react and each having common knowledge of the specifics of the mission.

In the comprehensive care setting, a team needs the same cohesiveness in its mission of treating, say, diabetes within the family setting. The team will need to define, specifically and uniquely for them, who is responsible and how best to handle (a) the patient's emotional state, (b) genetic counseling, (c) early screening and diagnosis, (d) treatment of acute episodes, (e) long-term management of the patient, and (f) patient education. Furthermore, the team will also need to have specific and unique answers to what should be done where (in the Center, in the hospital, in the home) and by whom.

One of the most significant findings in the MLK Health Center was that in many ways the center's educational strategy was subverting its managerial strategy. The primary goal of center management was to have effective teams delivering health care to the particular patient population. Therefore, effective team functioning was important. Much of the educational activity, however, was aimed at helping people learn about the work in situations which *maintained the integrity of their original roles.* Two examples:

1. Family health workers, upon entering the system, received six months or so of training in a class composed entirely of family health workers. Only afterwards did they join a team, where they were expected to be "instant" team members.
2. Internists might be teaching the same medical content to nurses on Tuesday, to family health workers on Wednesday, to doctors on Thursday. But application of this content to a patient could not be adequately discussed in that classroom setting since the *team* was the appropriate unit for discussing how to apply content to actual practice.

After recognizing the contradiction, a reorganization of educational programs and priorities was undertaken. The heads of services analyzed what content could and should be taught to the team as a team. It was assumed the application of what is learned would be most effective when the team itself could become a classroom or learning community.

Obviously it is not possible to teach everything in a team setting. However, an effective strategy might be to maximize rather than minimize what is taught in the team setting. Types of subject matter that can be taught in a team include clinical content, problem solving and communication skills, community diagnosis, and patient diagnosis.

Medical service heads in this center are working to become better acquainted with educational technology—teaching methods, learning designs, use of teaching aids, etc. For example, in teaching treatment of hypertension to teams, the learning design might look like this:

| *Subject Matter* | *Method* | *Who* |
|---|---|---|
| Basic theory | Lecture | Medical service chiefs |
| Application to community area | Discussion | Team leaders |
| Application to specific patient population | Analysis and cases | Teams |

The problem of transferring skills from one profession to another is a special subquestion that needs attention. In learning theory, for example, what is involved in transferring "knowledge" is the teacher telling and the student listening. This is quite different from what is involved in transferring "skill," where the student must *practice* the skill. In applying this principle to the transfer of competence from one role to another—for example, pediatrician to nurse—some studies have indicated that there are several gaps between what is apparently learned and what is in fact usable. Opportunities to practice skills in a controlled and supervised setting (such as an intern on a hospital ward) are limited in community medicine.

Furthermore, there tends to be a lag between learning a skill and being able to practice it under supervision. In a study of nurses, the fact emerged that the nurses felt competent to do only those things that they had learned in their basic nursing education, although they had been taught many other things in connection with their new roles. And they even felt relatively low competence in the skills they had learned on the job from the physicians.[2] In another study, a gap was shown to exist between those things that nurses indicated they felt competent to do and were authorized to do by physicians and the practices which they were in fact doing as perceived by patients and members of their health teams.[3]

On the basis of these findings, we can generalize in terms of educational strategy that:

1. Where people desire to become more "professional," there is a corrollary concern about not being as competent professionally as their teachers. This produces conservative behavior and a tendency not to practice newly learned skills. (Example: nurses who compared themselves to doctors did not use their authorized, newly acquired skills.)
2. The type of learning, e.g., knowledge or skill, should guide the particular educational method. (Example: skills cannot be learned from lectures; they must be practiced.)
3. The setting (the class) in which material is taught is perhaps the most important single variable. If application is required, the class should be those who have to apply the knowledge (in this case, the health teams). If skill is the goal, people with comparable backgrounds and preparation may compose a "best class." However, in each case the choice should be conscious.

## SOME SOCIAL ISSUES WITH ORGANIZATIONAL IMPLICATIONS

I want to touch briefly on three issues which I believe have important implications for managing comprehensive community-based health care. They are:

1. The effects of different backgrounds and reference groups on collaborative work.
2. The effects of "professionalism" on the carrying out of the work.
3. The effects of changing and different value systems on the people and the work.

**Effects of Different Backgrounds**

Look at the number and variety of backgrounds included in a comprehensive health care delivery team.

- Medical specialists (internists, pediatricians, psychiatrists, obstetricians, dentists).
- Physicians in their first or second year of residency.
- Interns in community medicine.
- Public health nurses with some special training.
- Community resident family health workers with six months of special training.
- Lawyers.
- Social workers and community development specialists.

When people from these very different backgrounds are asked to work as colleagues or peers, tension is produced. For example:

1. An internist trained in the traditional doctor-patient relationship may have real difficulty in "sharing" the patient with other health workers.
2. When public health nurses, trained in medical education and delivery of services, are asked to function as leaders of teams composed of doctors and other health workers, they find this role very difficult to perform.
3. Community health workers with no previous health care experience are expected to contribute to the diagnosis and treatment of patients. They find it most difficult to discuss, as colleagues, the information they have obtained about patients because they doubt their own competence as compared to the doctor's and nurse's.

The results of this tension are reduction in information flow, low-level compromise, little challenge of ideas, low trust, and lowering of commitment to get the job done.

A "businesslike approach" to the task will not, in itself, solve these problems. Administrators need to develop programs in which relevant groups such as health teams can talk about their difficulties and jointly work out methods of dealing with them.

**The Effects of Professionalism**

A question facing any organization composed of a variety of capabilities and professions is: To what degree do professional standards and ethics, professional loyalties, and the relationship between types of education and training required for accreditation affect the work. In traditional medical systems it is relatively clear by accreditation who is able to provide what care. For example, traditionally a physician does prenatal care. However, as we move more and more into team practice, the need to conserve the physician's resources for those things that *only* he can do requires that health workers with different backgrounds and accreditation begin to carry out some of the tasks that were formerly part of his job.

Relevant questions that then arise are: What are those things that *only* the accredited physician can and should do? Who should decide? What education, re-education, and accreditation is needed to have certain things done by persons other than physicians? Who should decide?

A related question involves rewards. When functions can be performed by people with varying degrees of training, education, and accreditation, what are the implications for their relative compensation? Their career possibilities? Their accreditation? More and more the issue of "professionalism" will be occupying administrators and health delivery institution managers.

Edgar Schein, in his book on professional education, has some relevant comments about this subject. He says:

> "The problem of definition derives from the fact that we are attempting to give precision to a social or occupational role that varies as a function of the setting within which it is performed, which is itself evolving, and which is perceived differently by different segments of society."[4]

I suspect this has important implications for community health care management.

**Effects of Changing Value Systems**

A major factor affecting the management of health care delivery in any setting—but especially in the community setting—is the multiple value systems found in both patient populations and the deliverers of care. As we move into an era of higher expectations and more social distance between the "haves" and "have nots"; as we experience stronger social pressure for egalitarianism from a number of minorities and see increasing concern with issues of life style, we find a new set of values expressed by many of the health workers emerging from medical and professional schools.

It has been my experience that younger men and women, more than their older counterparts, tend to focus on the social values of health care. For instance, there was a dramatic difference between some of the older doctors at the MLK Center and some of the younger physicians. The former saw the role of the medical practitioner as one of providing technically excellent care to all patients; the younger men were much more concerned with the social aspects of the delivery of health care to the community. They wanted to focus more effort on social action and helping community residents to take more responsibility for managing their own health care.

Certainly no community health care institution's administration can afford to ignore this changing mix of values on the part of practicing health workers, patient populations, and the communities in which they live. An analysis of the values of the subpopulations that comprise the system—patients and deliverers of health care—with explicit attention paid to this in management planning, is one likely organizational direction.

## IMPLICATIONS FOR THE EDUCATION OF HEALTH WORKERS

Based on my experience with the Dr. Martin Luther King, Jr. Health Center as well as discussions with various personnel in similar community-based delivery institutions, I believe that the education of physicians and other health workers who are moving into social and community medicine should include various managerial skills that are relevant to medical institutions.

There is a need today for capabilities in designing organization structures that promote the improved delivery of health care, competence in the management of decision making, team development, career development, information systems, community and organization development, and planning and managing change. Medical institutions also need to have both the capability for managing short-term work and that required for planning the organization of the future.

While I believe that training in such managerial skills should be built into the curricula of medical and nursing schools, in the short run we need to bring people into medical institutions who already have competence in these specialties. The management schools are one likely source for providing some of these near-term resources. More and more, graduates of business and industrial management programs have the knowledge and skills in organization development, psychology, information systems, and management methods that are needed to manage complex institutions. They also tend to have the kinds of social values required for effective functioning in a community setting. Therefore, these graduates might well become a source of talent for organization planning and perhaps for leadership in some medical institutions.

In the longer run, if we are to prepare health professionals for managing as well as providing the kinds of comprehensive health care we are discussing, the curricula in health sciences training institutions need to be developed or expanded in the following areas:

1. Social system theory and its application to organization.

2. Systems analysis.
3. Organizational behavior—the dynamics of organization, structural design, decision making.
4. Group dynamics, group development, and team building.
5. Leadership and supervisory training.
6. Information systems management.
7. The process and planning of change.
8. Interpersonal and communication skills.

While some of this content is already included in the curricula of certain medical and other professional schools, the point I want to emphasize is the need for more such content. These matters should receive the joint attention of heads of medical schools, administrators of teaching hospitals, and directors of community health centers.

## SUMMARY

Toward the goal of achieving more effective management of team delivery of health care, I have examined some of the organizational problems involved in the management of comprehensive family-based ambulatory care in the community setting. Hopefully, I have demonstrated that a body of knowledge exists in the behavioral and management sciences today relating to the management of complex organizations which, I firmly believe, can and should be used to help medical institutions deal with the constellation of problems outlined in this chapter.

The present separation of the profession of medicine from the field of management will, I hope, be more a matter of historical record than of future reality. A merger of these capabilities, one can only conclude from the evidence, would not only be in the best interests of both fields, but, above this, in the best interests of our society as a whole.

## NOTES

1. My convictions developed principally through working with the director and management staff of the MLK Center in the South Bronx in New York City. During the time covered in this chapter the center, which is part of Montefiore Hospital, was under the direction of Dr. Harold Wise.
2. "Factors Influencing the Expansion of the Nurse's Role in the Primary Care Setting: A Study of the Graduates of a Nurse Practitioner Program," by Mark S. Gerstein and Eric L. Herzog with Drs. Ann S. Baker and Stephen E. Goldfinger, Sloan School of Management Working Paper #639–73, January 1973, 50 Memorial Drive, Cambridge, Mass. 02139.

3. "Role Satisfaction of Public Health Nurses on Health Care Teams" by Regina C. McCormack, M.D. Unpublished paper, Dr. Martin Luther King, Jr. Health Center, 3674 Third Avenue, Bronx, New York 10456.
4. E. Schein, *Professional Education: Some New Directions.* Prepared by the Sloan School of Management, MIT, for the Carnegie Commission on The Future of Higher Education, 1971.

## A SPECIAL NOTE

An earlier version of this chapter appeared as an article in the *Milbank Quarterly,* July 1972; Part I, Vol. 50.

Appendix

# Evaluation of Team Effectiveness as it Relates to Patient Care

*Richard Beckhard*

Evaluation of team effectiveness involves a number of sticky questions which nonetheless need to be addressed. For example, have we any proof that teams whose members work well together are more effective in delivering patient care than teams whose members don't work well together? What are realistic measures of productivity? What, indeed, is an effective team? And what assumptions, if any, can be made about the relationship between high morale and effective work? Let us attempt to address each of these questions.

First, the relationship between increased team effectiveness and better patient care. We have not, as yet, any valid measures which prove that patients actually receive better care from a more effective team as opposed to a less effective one. However, there is evidence that the teams in the MLK Center are, in fact, now providing the same or better quality of care than they were before the early MIT interventions, even though they have almost doubled the number of patient families they serve. But the evidence is quantitative, and we do not feel such measures are the truly relevant ones to "prove" this relationship.

Yet we do make some assumptions about better care as related to team behavior that can be measured. Some examples follow.

> If a health delivery team is *consciously* and *continuously* looking at its own resources to see how to optimize them in delivering patient care, we postulate that it will provide better care than a team that is not doing this.

Evidence shows that, after training, the MLK teams were better able to consciously assess their resources and to reallocate some tasks. For example, physicians were able to turn over to family health workers and nurses some of the work they previously had done on their own. Team members were also better able to coordinate certain delivery functions. The treatment of hypertension and diabetes, for example, was restructured to include the resources supplied by a family health worker making a home visit rather than relying entirely on the physician who sees the patient in the examining room. These new treatment modes were designed to make use of the contributions that various health team members could make.

> If a health delivery team is *consciously* and *continuously* building a feedback system from patients in terms of what patients hear, remember, and use; in terms of their own health management; and in terms of patients' reports of their attitudes toward health care, we postulate that this team would be delivering better patient care.

There is some evidence that this activity increased after the MLK teams' OD training. Some of the health teams built specific feedback systems into their work; some teams made studies of the people in the geographical area they served. One major feedback system that showed improvement was the team conference; information held by individual team members, which had previously gone unreported, was now shared with the rest of the team. Such sharing resulted in changed procedures and, we postulate, better patient care.

> If health delivery teams are able to get their own "house in order" regarding decision making, communication procedures, meeting individual needs, clarifying roles, etc., we postulate that they will have more energy to put into patient care, because less energy will be needed for team maintenance and coping with members' interpersonal problems.

The evidence clearly supports the fact that training in more adequate decision making, clearer role perceptions and expectations, more openness in communications, and a conscious effort to establish more functional norms resulted in more energy being available for the common task of providing patient care. Significantly, there was a high correlation between the team's ability to direct energy toward patient care and a common understanding of the goals and their priorities as they related to the specific work to be done by different members of the team.

Now let us look at questions two and three. What are some realistic measures of productivity? And what is an effective team? We submit that productivity and team effectiveness can be measured along the dimensions listed below.

> **Clarity of objectives and mission:** Agreement on the team's objectives and mission should be shared by all team members. Agreement should also be reached on the priorities assigned to multiple objectives.

**"Good" decision making and problem solving processes:** All team members need to develop problem solving skills. These include the ability to look at a problem systematically and analytically; the ability to collect the appropriate facts; the ability to adequately define the problem; the ability to generate alternative solutions; and, finally, the ability to make use of all of these factors to arrive at a "best" decision, which automatically means one that is supported by all team members.

**Clear role expectations:** Open discussion leading to an understanding of the core functions of the roles of physicians, nurses, family health workers, and any other health workers connected with the team is critical to team effectiveness. For example, a core aspect of the family health worker's role is patient management and ongoing contact with the patient; education and regular preventive treatment is a key part of the nurse's role; diagnosis and treatment of acute illness is a major aspect of the doctor's role. Beyond this it is necessary to explicitly define where any of these roles overlap in terms of any particular patient. Realistic expectations on the part of each team member as to what other members can contribute is also critical. How the team handles these various aspects of role will tell us a good deal about the team's effectiveness.

**Norms that support the task:** Ground rules are needed that help team members achieve their objective of good patient care. For example, a team norm that requires all team members to share whatever information they have on a patient family rather than withholding it for personal reasons is critical to good patient care. Norms that allow people to share with other team members their anxieties and concerns about their adequacy to perform certain functions are also helpful in getting the team's task accomplished. Norms that reward members for directing most of their energy toward patient care are also functional.

**Concern for each other's needs:** This may seem to contradict the previous statement but to the degree that there is a norm of concern for each team member's needs, the team is able to function more effectively and more energy is therefore available for patient care.

**Optimizing resources for growth and enlarging individual jobs:**
To the degree that the team can make use of its various resources to enlarge and/or enrich the jobs of team members, team functioning as a whole will be enhanced. For example, the physician who takes time to teach other team members certain clinical procedures and skills, or the family health worker who keeps doctors and nurses informed about the community's priorities, prejudices, and social

values is each contributing to the effectiveness of other team members and therefore to the team as a whole.

Finally, what assumptions can be made about the relationship of high morale and good feelings to effective work? Let us state immediately that high morale does not necessarily lead to high productivity. The goals of a team improvement effort are greater productivity and increased motivation toward improved task performance—not high morale per se. Happiness and feelings of comfort, while desirable, are not possible at all times nor are they a necessary condition for achieving high productivity. However, satisfaction derived from achieving task goals does have a high correlation with productivity.

In sum, one may say that although it is not yet possible (and perhaps never will be) to prove a specific correlation between the effectiveness of a team's internal functioning and the effectiveness of the delivery of health care to patients, we submit that it is possible, in a broad sense, to measure and therefore to improve the effectiveness of a team's functioning by helping the team move toward the optimum end of the scale on the dimensions we have briefly outlined here.

## About Chapter Four

*Every organization, like every individual, theoretically at least, would like to be self-renewing. To possess this quality would not only insure continued responsiveness and flexibility but would also go far toward avoiding the pitfalls associated with rigidity and aging.*

*Yet often, both on the organizational and individual levels, little is done to achieve this desirable state, even though methods exist to promote just such qualities as innovativeness and flexibility.*

*At the MLK Center, where innovative responses to a demanding environment are critically important to the work of the agency, building an internal OD capability made good sense, particularly in late 1971. The reasoning was that if the center had a group of people trained as OD facilitators, they could continue to build on the work already done with the MIT consultants.*

*So it was that in December of that year a small group of MLK employees gathered in the deputy project director's office to hear the MIT people describe a training program designed to help them develop OD intervention and consultation skills. The mood that day was one of cautious enthusiasm.*

*In Chapter Four, the training program is described from the point of view of one of the participants. Not only did the 80 odd hours of work over a period of some five months require a high level of commitment to the training but also a capacity to tolerate large doses of frustration, confusion, and feelings of inadequacy. The question kept arising: How could these skills be mastered in such a short time? How could the trainees become effective consultants in only five months? Yet from management's vantage the questions were the opposite: What's taking so long? When are these people going to do something useful for MLK?*

*In the following chapter, Aileen Kyte points out that the problems arising from management's lack of understanding of what such a training program involves can jeopardize the effort to build an internal OD capability. Yet understanding in itself is not enough. In a real sense, management too needs to be trained in how to effectively utilize this new resource. Only then, by combining the newly acquired skills of both groups, is the organization likely to move toward the goal of becoming self-renewing.*

Chapter Four

# Creating a Self-Renewing Capability: An OD Odyssey

*Aileen L. Kyte*

## PART I—THE CONCEPT

Back in the early days of the MLK Center, Ron Brooke, the first research direc-
or, peddled a dream. Every employee, he said, from the project director down
o the security guard should be a healer. The whole center, he believed, should
e permeated with the healing concept. Since it was hard to find medical people,
et alone others, who thought in such terms, the dream remained a dream. The
ools to make it a reality were not at hand.

While a self-renewing organization is not exactly the stuff from which Ron Brooke fashioned his dream, it is concerned with creating a system that en-
courages individual self-development and growth within the framework of carry-
ng out an organization's objectives and goals.

In the fall of 1971, MLK's management began to consider what next
teps would be most useful in moving toward this goal of achieving a self-renewing
organization. At this point the MIT consultants had already worked with six of
he eight health care delivery teams and with the agency's overall administrative
tructure. Now the question was: How could the center build an internal OD cap-
bility that would help to ensure that MLK would become a truly self-renewing
organization?

In a series of meetings that fall involving MIT's Irv Rubin, the three
op MLK managers—Bill Lloyd, Deloris Smith, Ed Martin—and Harold Wise, a
trategy was hammered out in the form of a two-pronged effort. First, to meet
he agency's pressing need for middle management training (some 30 people had
ecently been promoted from the ranks to supervisory level responsibilities),
MIT would help MLK's training department to plan and implement a program
or these people, utilizing OD techniques. Although initially it would involve
only ten people, later the training would be made available to all middle
managers.

The second part of the plan was in some ways more ambitious. A cross section of agency personnel would be selected for training as internal OD change agents, with the deputy project director acting as chairman of this effort.

While the primary goal was to build an internal OD capability, an immediate impetus behind this program, at least in terms of management's thinking, was a planned organizational change involving the health teams. Instead of the loosely structured twelve-or-so member team, management wanted to formalize a smaller unit, called a basic work team or BWT. The BWT unit would comprise four persons: family health worker, public health nurse, internist, and pediatrician—all of whom, at least theoretically, would be involved in managing a family's health care. In fact, such an arrangement already operated informally on some teams.

The thinking here was that this smaller, more closely knit unit could substantially increase the quality and quantity of health care delivered to client families. The BWT, management reasoned, would not only lessen the communications problems so often found on the larger teams, but would also provide for a clarification of each person's role that was not presently being achieved.

The BWT strategy also involved the changed position of the family health worker, who had only recently been made responsible for developing and coordinating a comprehensive health plan for each of her 100 to 200 families—a task which had previously been part of the nurse's responsibility. To accomplish this, the family health worker was supposed to have the assistance of the nurse, internist, and pediatrician. On paper at least, this seemed to mean that the pyramid was to be set on its head: rather than low man on the totem pole, the family health worker would now be on top, with doctors and nurses acting as staff to her line authority.

The first real life assignment of the OD trainees would be to assist in the implementation of the basic work team concept on an experimental basis with selected teams. This, it was felt, would not only help management implement the desired change but would also provide the trainees with a fairly structured, clear-cut situation for their first intervention. The training itself would take some 80 hours of work with the MIT consultants over a period of about five months. It would cover pretty much the same ground as a year's training in the Sloan School program at MIT in Cambridge.

## PART II—THE TRAINING

Before I attempt to describe the training process that was used to develop an internal OD capability at the Dr. Martin Luther King, Jr. Health Center, let me caution the reader that what follows in Part II constitutes one member's experience in such a training program. It is my story of the group's odyssey; no one else in that group, or certainly in any other group, had exactly the same experience. Each person's experience is uniquely his or her own.

Yet most members of experiential groups go through almost predictable periods of frustration, anger, confusion—and insight; of good feelings and bad feelings; of getting it all together only to have it fall apart Humpty Dumpty fashion; of somehow picking up the pieces and trying once again. And, finally, of making connections between the experiences and the conceptual material related to them; of then making the whole of it part of oneself.

Because of this commonality of experience in such training groups; because of the general lack of recognition on the part of most managements of the time, energy, and emotion involved; and—critically important—because of the consequences likely to result from such a lack of understanding, we feel it is useful to describe in some detail both the content and the process of OD training at the MLK Center.

In what follows, bowing to the convention of the day, I have not used last names. Instead, group members were asked to select whatever name they wanted to have used in this description of our training. Interestingly, more than half wanted their own names used. Trainers' names are also their own.

### Great Expectations

On a gray day in early December of 1971, sixteen people had been summoned to a meeting in the deputy project director's office. Irv Rubin and Mark Plovnick from MIT, plus the people selected for training and a few guests, sat crowded in the smallish room. Each of the prospective trainees had received the following memo:

> In order to build upon and extend the effectiveness of the team building program run by the MIT group during the spring and summer, we have decided to develop within the agency our own intervention capabilities.
>
> In collaboration with the MIT group, we will train some people from different areas of the agency as "intervenors." We would appreciate your participation in this effort. Your involvement in this effort has been approved by your department head.
>
> Mrs. Valerie M., deputy project director, will be the chairman of this training effort.

This was the extent of the MLK employees' knowledge of why they had been asked to attend the meeting that day.

I arrived at this meeting via a different route. Since I was compiling a history of the OD effort at MLK, Harold Wise suggested I sit in. Three or four faces were familiar to me as I entered Valerie M's office; the rest were strangers. After brief around-the-room introductions, Valerie outlined the criteria that had been used to select agency employees for OD training. Briefly they were:

1. People from the community or having intimate knowledge of it.
2. Commitment to the agency and its goals.
3. Knowledge of the agency.
4. Acceptability to others in the agency; high level of trust with others.

5. A representative slice of the agency.
6. Ability to listen and work with people.

On the basis of these criteria, twelve persons had been selected for the OD training group. Besides the deputy project director, they included the head of training, head of operations analysis, the chief internist, two members of the social medicine internship and residency program, the director of allied health services, the medical records supervisor, a family health worker, a public health nurse, a member of the community health advocacy department, and a medical services administration representative. Four out of this group of twelve had been involved in the earlier MIT team interventions.

Irv Rubin, who would be one of the trainers in the weeks ahead (Mark Plovnick was the other), then took over the meeting. Irv, young, intense, buoyant, with a flair for the dramatic, offered up some heady fare that afternoon. We would learn exciting new skills—and very marketable ones. We were to begin thinking of ourselves as a new department at MLK. We would have a library at our disposal and a room would be reserved for OD activities. Some of us might well go on to new careers in this field, acting not only as consultants to MLK but also to other health centers and related organizations. Although more than 30 people had been considered for this program, we were the chosen few. While each person would continue to function in his/her job during the training, top management had not only agreed to make time available for the training sessions but also for at least some of the homework assignments we would be expected to do.

The training would initially focus, Irv said, on group process and group dynamics. We would then examine the process of organizational change and the helping relationship. Finally we would look at various intervention models which would culminate in an actual intervention.

Now, were there any questions? Was there anyone who didn't feel he or she could take on the responsibility involved in this important assignment? It was very quiet in the room. Finally the questions started. What will happen to my regular work assignments? Who will cover for me on my job? What happens to my patients? Where is the time coming from—we can't get everything done as it is! And then—What makes you feel I can do this kind of work? I'm not sure I even understand what it is.

"That's what the training is all about," Irv said confidently.

A little later an around-the-room check underscored the reservations but no one asked for out. "If the deputy project director thinks I can do this, then at least I'll give it a try," summed up several responses. (Perhaps, I thought, the distance from a health center in the South Bronx to the Massachusetts Institute of Technology in Cambridge would turn out to be a negotiable trip.)

Before the meeting could be adjourned we had to decide on four days in January for our initial training sessions. A two-day weekend retreat, away from family and job responsibilities, Irv said, would be the best way to begin. Startled looks. A whole weekend? Away? We settled for two nine-to-five, back-to-back sessions, on Friday, January 7, and Saturday, January 8, with full days also scheduled for January 18 and 21. We'd meet at the Moses Library at Montefiore.

"How do we get there?" someone asked, looking at the deputy project director. "Can we have a car from the center take us over?" Yes, she could arrange that; those needing transportation would meet in the MLK lobby at 8:30 Friday morning. "What about Saturday morning?" someone else asked. "I'll have to check that out," said Valerie M. Her look seemed to imply: It shouldn't be that hard for you to get over to Moses on your own.

A word about the deputy project director and the chairman of our group. One of the first "core" trainees in the agency, she had moved up the MLK hierarchy from family health worker to her present position in less than four years, and was living proof of the agency's commitment to bring community people into top management positions. A big, powerful woman with almost blue-black skin, a razor sharp mind, mother of seven, Valerie M. had her own brand of charisma. She also had little patience with those of us who moved at a slower pace. What would her role as chairman of this training effort be in the weeks and months ahead, I wondered.

### The Days at Moses Library

It was bitterly cold that Friday morning in January when we assembled in the Moses Library, a large, book-lined, carpeted room—real luxury compared to the MLK facilities. Coffee and Danish had been ordered and we talked inconsequentially as we waited for latecomers to arrive. The group provided with the MLK car were the last to show.

Now we could begin. Was anyone else as tense as I? I looked around the room at the circle of faces. Everyone seemed to be wearing a mask. What was behind those masks, I wondered. My own, I knew, tried to cover the anxious question of whether I, an outsider, would be accepted by the group. I had already sensed that Irv was surprised and not pleased to see me here. Well, the final decision, I suspected, would rest with the group.

Irv was talking now. We were here, he said, to learn organization development skills, which we would use as third party intervenors or change agents. While the emphasis would be on experiential learning, there would also be related conceptual material which we would be expected to read. However, our learning would be primarily in the group itself. And it would be up to us to decide what kind of group we were going to be—a theme that would be repeated many times in the weeks to come.

Now an around-the-circle check to see where each of us was and what we expected to get out of the training. For the next hour or so, as people spoke up hesitantly, I sat frozen. Why, I thought, should it be so important to me to be in this group? I'd been in lots of groups—as participant, as trainer; if they didn't accept me, so what? Finally, in a voice I hardly recognized, I broke into an exchange between Al W. and Dr. C. I said I was feeling terribly anxious—that I didn't know if the group would let me in.

"Why *are* you here?" I heard Irv asking.

Defensively I answered, "Well, Harold told me to come." Then I added, "I see it as a real opportunity to learn more about both OD and MLK."

"That last part makes me feel more comfortable," I heard Mark Plovnick say. Then two or three people in the group came to my defense. I began to relax. But Irv wasn't finished. "My first priority is the MLK people; if it comes to a crunch my choice will have to be with them. Can you live with that situation?"

"I don't know," I answered, "I guess I want to try."

Somehow I felt I'd already paid my membership dues in this group. Even though I remained partly the outsider, I wanted to stay.

### Emphasis on Experiential

Experiential learning, we all found out very quickly if we didn't already know, meant, literally, *experiencing.* No one, our trainers pointed out, expects to learn to ride a bicycle or drive a car or swim or play tennis or cook by simply reading books on the subjects. The learning comes by doing.

So it would be with us. We would learn by doing, by experiencing—ourselves, each other, the dynamics of our interactions. While in the traditional T group situation this could mean letting the group develop its own experiences with no agenda provided, in our case we would learn by doing a series of tasks or exercises designed to help us understand key OD concepts and develop our skills as third party intervenors. In the process, we would cooperate; we would compete; we would try to learn to give constructive feedback, and in turn to use the feedback we were given constructively; we would experience dependency and what is involved in being responsible for a dependent person. We would learn about contract negotiation with a client, data collection and feedback, and intervention models. We would work in pairs, in triads, and in learning groups outside the training sessions. We would know failure and, once in a while, success. All this and much more would be involved in the exercises that were to be the core of our experiential training in the weeks ahead.

While I will describe some of these learning experiences here, my primary focus will be on the group as it moved from an agglomeration of individuals to an interdependent group with a mission. Not an easy journey for anyone; not all of us who started that Friday morning would stay the distance.

### The Competitive Drive

Being in a good experiential learning group is a little like riding a roller coaster. It's exciting, a little frightening, it knocks the breath out of you, and before you can collect yourself, you're into another nose dive.

The first days of our training felt something like that. We did so much; we tried so hard; we failed so often. And we also learned. Take our decision making exercise on the first day at Moses. Group decision making–no big deal. For this particular task we were divided into two subgroups, As and Bs. The As' task was to select one out of eleven given alternatives to a complex (and basically unsolvable) problem, within a time limit of 30 minutes. While the As worked, the Bs were to observe how they went about their task.

Group A members were polite as they grappled with their problem. They listened to each other, even when points seemed irrelevant or people long-winded. There was relatively little interrupting and no voices were raised. They were still struggling to define the task when Irv called time.

"Time?"

"Already?"

No one had been checking on the time.

As the As moved to the outer circle, the Bs moved to the center and the process was reversed. Although not put in words, clearly the Bs felt they could do better with a similar problem they had been given. A timekeeper was immediately appointed to inform the group as each five minutes passed. A task oriented minority resolutely pushed for consensus–almost any consensus–just so we reached a decision. Under less-than-gentle prodding, dissatisfied members gave way. A little before the 30 minutes were up we had our decision.

Our elation was short-lived.

"Okay, you've gotten your decision," said Irv. "Now let's check your commitment to it." On a scale of one (no commitment) to seven (total commitment) each of us was asked to indicate his/her level of commitment to the decision. The answers clustered around one and two.

"You'd be in trouble if you had to implement that decision," Irv remarked wryly.

Now the As were elated. The Bs, too, it seemed, had failed.

Hard to win any Brownie points around here, I thought.

Mark and Irv were saying, "Now let's look at the process of what just happened." Our behavior, it seemed, was almost classic. Group A had paid attention to member needs (no attempt to halt off-target excursions, no interrupting, etc.) but had lost sight of the assigned task. Group B, on the other hand, under strong competitive pressures to beat the As, had focussed on task and neglected member needs. The dual components of getting the task done and paying attention to individual needs, Irv pointed out, requires a delicate balance–a balance that shifts with the particular circumstances and problem at hand.

As we sat glumly, Mark said, "Nobody really wins or loses in these exercises. But hopefully everybody learns."

We began to feel better.

When we did our around-the-circle check before breaking at five, the consensus was it had been a good day, a good beginning. We felt tired yet exhilarated. Could it really have been only eight hours ago that many of these people had been strangers to me? On the subway going downtown, I treid to sort out the impressions that crowded in on each other. It's a good group, I thought; I'm glad I'm in it.

When we assembled at nine the next morning we felt like old friends who had shared some important experience. The tension that had marked yesterday morning was gone—although, as we would learn, that was a temporary phenomenon. The roller coaster was soon in motion again.

### Anatomy of a Trainer

By the end of January, our experience-based learning had covered such subjects as perceptions and stereotyping, giving and receiving feedback, styles of leadership, theories of helping and the helping relationship, conflict resolution, and the use of a force field analysis.

Not all the exercises we undertook were uniformly successful. In some we got bogged down and bored; in some we failed to make connections between the task we were doing (the experience) and the conceptual material related to it. Indeed, the linking of the experiential and conceptual proved to be one of our greatest problems.

With all our ups and downs in the process of working together, we began to appreciate the capabilities that each of us brought to the group as well as the complementary skills of our trainers, Irv and Mark. Irv I have already briefly described—energetic, enthusiastic, direct, sometimes even cutting in his approach. Mark was younger, quieter, still in the process of completing his Ph.D. at MIT. As our sessions progressed I began to think of Mark as the "mender." When Irv had let the group have it, so to speak, Mark, with a quiet comment, an insightful question, would help us pick up the pieces and try again.

Their different personalities and approaches provided a graphic demonstration that trainers need not be cut out of the same cloth. The commonality they share is a set of values. These values, to which I would return many times as the training progressed, were outlined in our first reading assignment. "Good trainers," Matthew Miles wrote, "can be aggressive or docile, outgoing or reserved jovial or serious—but the trainer's personality must almost certainly include some commitment to norms such as the following:

> *People are important.* The trainer has a basic feeling of respect for the worth of persons. He does not interrupt, he listens; he rejects ideas but not people; he shows that he believes that persons are ends and all else is means. As he demonstrates his belief, he serves to some degree as a model for other group members, and the norm of basic respect for persons gradually becomes established in the training group.
>
> *It's safe to try things out here.* The trainer also indicates by his

actions that things are off the record in this group, that trying something new is not only permissible but desirable. He permits and invites discussion of his own behavior. He does not criticize anyone for expressing any feeling or idea. Gradually, willingness to experiment becomes a group norm too.

*Feelings are important.* The trainer takes expressions of feeling seriously. When people say they feel mad, sad, bad, glad, he helps the group see that these are basic data from which to work. Feelings of group members tell us how well progress on the task is going—whether people are interested and involved, whether the goal is clear, how well a particular leader's approach is working. Frank expression of feeling is essential if the group members are to understand the processes going on.

*Things are not taken personally.* The trainer responds objectively to expressions of feeling. Feelings are facts, his behavior says to the group. If Joe gets mad at me, that tells us something about what has been happening. From this we can learn about what leads to what in a group. Antagonism or syrupy smoothings-over have no place in what the trainer does. Too, when he encourages analysis of process, using a tape recorder, a process observer, or post-meeting reaction sheets, the trainer is in effect saying, "We can look at ourselves objectively and learn from this." As the group moves along, members come to share a work-centered kind of objectivity.

*We learn from doing things and analyzing them.* From the start, the trainer indicates by his actions that he sees learning as beginning with concrete experience. He does not lecture the group, and he does not encourage windy discussions of "leadership" or "how to handle the blocker." He helps the group members examine their own experience. He helps them set up trials of particular approaches to problems. He helps the group members think about what they have done. More and more as the training group proceeds, the members act as if they too shared this basic norm—that provisional trials, carefully analyzed, are the major road to learning.

*What's happening here and now is the important thing.* The trainer does not usually encourage the group members to talk about the past, other groups, back-home experiences, things they have read, or what might happen in the future. Mostly, he talks directly to what is going on in the training group as it is happening right now, right here. By what he says and does he dramatizes his belief that the problem is not someone else's behavior, but our own behavior as it is unfolding every minute in front of our own eyes.

*We plan together.* Finally, the trainer shows the group members that he believes the training group is basically a shared, planful enterprise. He does not spring things on the group. He does not attempt to pull his rank on others. He does not take a laissez-faire attitude; he invites cooperative planning. He refuses to take sole responsibility for the success of the training group.[1]

Miles concludes that it is far more important that the trainer accept these norms as part of his personal value system than that he be especially proficient in specific methods and techniques of training.

Little doubt that our trainers were committed to OD values. And little doubt that we as a group were committed to learning OD skills, to improving our capabilities as intervenors and change agents. But our commitment to each other, to the group—how did we really feel about that? How far were we willing to go? This would be tested in terms of some of the problems the group already was facing.

**Pressing Problems**

Since this group had been selected as a microcosm of the agency, as such it presented many of the problems besetting MLK. There was one problem, however, that I saw no sign of in all the group's time together: racial tensions, particularly black vs. Puerto Rican, which had often surfaced in MLK, did not affect us. Our skin color, which ranged from black to rich olive to white, was not a problem.

However, just as in the center, we did have serious difficulties relating to time and work pressures: people came late, had to leave early, even missed whole sessions. Telephone and beeper interruptions often made us feel that the training was not being given a top priority as promised. Sometimes homework assignments (which proved to take much more time than anyone expected) were not completed or not done at all. This at times led to sharp exchanges between those who had done the work and those who hadn't. We had trouble working out dates for our "between" meetings as well as for the February training sessions with Mark and Irv.

We also had our share of the problems that face any vertical-slice group of an organization. Position in the MLK hierarchy affected behavior in our group in many ways. Were doctors "more equal" than other members? Did department heads have an edge on subordinate employees? Who went to lunch with whom? Would everyone be called by his/her first name—including doctors? Was Valerie M, as chairman of this training program and deputy project director, a member like everyone else, or was her role different? In one of the first sessions she had spoken briefly of her own problems in this area. The response was: "We're all in this together; the MLK hierarchy should not determine our roles in this group." Easily said; not so easily achieved.

Sometimes Valerie seemed to be with us, and we all felt better; sometimes she seemed to be somewhere else and a tension went through the group. Gladys V., Ann S., and Eleanor M. said, in effect, "Come in Valerie, we need you." But these attempts to draw her in were never completely successful. When I asked, "Where are you at, Valerie?" as we reassembled after lunch one day, her response was an enigmatic look. It wouldn't be until after our formal training had ended late in May that Valerie, in a long taped interview, would answer my question.

Valerie was not the only person to have a role problem in the OD group. Maria R., head of training and one of Harold Wise's original top team members, was also in a difficult spot. Did her training expertise, for instance, mean that she was expected to be an expert in this group? Did her seniority at the center set her apart from others?

Maria talked a lot. Sometimes I felt her words were like layers of protective coating. One day in a sharp exchange with another group member, Maria suddenly became quiet. Then she started to cry. As Irv crossed the room to comfort her, I also moved to Maria's side. I felt other group members pull back. Such emotionalism, they seemed to be saying, is out of bounds. What if everybody in the group started to cry? How would we get our work done?

*"Feelings are facts; they are part of the data we work with."* It was a statement we had all read in our assignments. But in this task-oriented group we had great difficulty dealing with feelings; they were never accorded the respectability of the so-called hard data.

With all our problems I think Ann S., the public health nurse, summed up the group's attitude in the early stages of the training; after looking intently around the circle one afternoon, she said, "I like everybody here. There's no one I don't like in this group."

Our last session in January was a highpoint for us—and would remain that for a long time to come. We were to view a screening of "Twelve Angry Men" and try to relate the jury's attempt to reach a decision to the group process concepts we were studying. Maybe it was the lack of tension, the fact that we weren't in competition with each other, the feeling it was not a regular work session. Whatever, a kind of euphoria spread through the group. It was safe to express feelings regarding the actors who peopled the film that we would not express toward each other. Perhaps it was our sense of openness that made us all feel like pros that day.

Early in February we lost our first member—Dr. C., chief internist and the only full-time MLK physician in the OD group. Dr. C. had voiced reservations about the training from the beginning. He was skeptical that inexperienced people could learn OD intervention skills in a relatively short training program. Also his commitment to his patients had put extra pressure on him—sometimes he had to leave early or he would be called away on an emergency in mid session.

That particular day we were well into a discussion of group norms, with Mark at the blackboard outlining some principles, when Dr. C. walked in. Perhaps he stayed twenty minutes; then he left, not saying anything. Mark promised to see him after the session, but I think we all knew he had decided to pull out. "I wish he had told the group," I said. "I feel it's a group failure, that we didn't care enough about keeping him." The looks and silence seemed to say: A doctor makes up his own mind; we don't have any influence on what Dr. C. does.

**Space Craft Enterprise**

We pushed on with our tasks, which were becoming more complicated, more difficult, and more directly related to what we would face in our first real intervention. In early February a four-hour simulation on planned change divided the group into members of the Enterprise Corp., which manufactured space craft, and the Merger Corp., a conglomerate which had just acquired Enterprise and would provide consulting help to that company. Our assignment was to read a 28-page article on planned change, which included instructions for the game we were to play. Those of us in Enterprise also received a sheet of specially lined paper, with six stars and the word Enterprise appearing twice. When this sheet was folded according to instructions, it became our finished product—a paper airplane. Our job was to organize ourselves to produce the largest possible profit, based on the number of planes we could make in five minutes of production time. All our materials (sheets of paper) had to be ordered in the 20-minute planning session that preceded making the planes. And we would lose money on any materials we didn't use.

The night before this session I sat up in bed rereading the instructions and familiarizing myself with the eleven-step procedure for folding the plane. After some practicing, using my kitchen timer, I found I could fold one plane a minute. I looked at the clock. It was after one. Ridiculous, I muttered; I'd been working on this silly exercise for almost three hours.

When Enterprise members met in Room 402 the next afternoon, we immediately faced problems. Dena S. had missed the previous session and had not gotten the assignment. Should we take the time now to help her learn the folding process or let her get along on her own as best she could? Valerie had spent several hours on the homework but announced she could not do the last part of the folding. Should one of us instruct her on the final steps or should her incomplete work be turned over to someone else to finish? Dave L. wanted to start by electing a president. Oh no, I thought, not that. I made a sample plane and handed it to Mark, our game coordinator. "Does this pass inspection?" I asked. After checking for quality control points, he nodded. Now the others were folding and checking their time. Quickly we figured that our team could complete 22 planes in five minutes, and on that basis we ordered our supply of materials. Then Mark called time and we started our production run.

It was incredible how tense it was. My fingers were suddenly all thumbs, my hands were shaking. I'd never finish five planes at this rate. Damn! I thought, I'd left my own feelings of anxiety out of my calculations when I figured on one plane a minute—and that omitted fact reduced my production by a third. Others also were falling behind. Between a high reject rate and the unused material we'd bought, we were deep in the red when the production run was over.

Now it was Merger's turn, as a consulting team, to help us improve our performance and our profits. After huddling for a few minutes, as we sat by stonily, Merger read off their suggestions. Their tone was condescending; their advice didn't seem to relate to what had happened. The Enterprise people were getting angrier. Some consultants—we needed them like a hole in the head! In our second production run, although we ordered less material, we lost more money.

When the "game" was finished, the book says we did a force-field analysis to help us better understand the process of change as it occurred in Merger's attempts to assist Enterprise. What I remember is the sound of the El trains rumbling by Room 402's windows in shortening intervals as the rush hour approached, and several of us grabbing our planes and hurling them across the room. "I made better planes than that when I was six years old," said Valerie as one nose-dived into the corner. "Whoever designed them should have his head examined."

When I got home that night I poured myself a stiff drink. A lot had happened that afternoon, but what did it have to do with planned change? I couldn't seem to sort it out or get it together. The very degree of my involvement in the exercise, it seemed, had made it impossible for me to really listen to what Irv and Mark had to say when the game was over. Indeed, it was several days before I stopped seeing group members as either Enterprise or Merger.

### Dependency and Self-Doubt

About this time in early February I began to sense a change taking place within the group. It was as though the more we learned and the closer we came to moving out into our first real intervention, the more we doubted ourselves and the more dependent we became on Irv and Mark. And the more we doubted our own capabilities, the more we questioned how realistic it was to think that within a period of weeks we would be competent to take on such an assignment. The distance from where we were and where Irv and Mark stood had never loomed greater.

Our self-doubts affected us in many ways. For one, our early sessions without Irv and Mark had been reasonably productive as we worked on assignments which would then be brought back to the next regular training session. Now these "between" sessions had deteriorated noticeably. People talked at the same time. No one seemed to listen any more. The feeling behind this behavior seemed to be: What did any of us really know that was worth listening to? Listening was now reserved for Irv's and Mark's pronouncements.

Our goodwill also diminished. We argued, we bickered, we fussed over trifles, and, it seemed to me, we scapegoated. After one of these sessions around this time I remember thinking, "Before the training started, I thought I knew something about OD. Now I don't know anything. It's all a big glob in my head."

Despite these negatives, we worked hard to prepare for the role play session scheduled for February 18. In this exercise we would explore the nature of entry into a client system and setting the initial contract with a client—two important segments of the model we would use in our first intervention that was coming upon us so fast.

The Friday afternoon of the role play we met in the Community Health Advocacy offices located in the Claremont Housing project in a long narrow room with kitchen facilities along one wall. A long table left barely enough room for the chairs surrounding it.

Group B was scheduled to play the client role first. As such we were divided into dentists and dental assistants, who in real life had been plagued with departmental problems. In the role play, the dental group had sent a memo to the internal OD group asking them to sit in on their next staff meeting to help them solve some of their more pressing problems.

As we squeezed into our chairs around the table, we noted that America, Gladys, and Ann, who had arrived early, were busy talking in whispers at one end of the room; other group A people did not seem to be involved.

America opened the role play by ringing up Valerie on an imaginary telephone and confirming the OD group's intention to attend the dental department's meeting, which in the role play would follow directly.

It didn't take long for the Bs to warm to the task of dentists vs. dental assistants. Frustration, anger, hurt all came pouring out. The attempts of our consultants to provide help were, in the main, ignored or rejected. Setting a contract with us that day was not in the cards.

When the role play was over I think Bs as well as As were shaken by what had happened. Did the Bs really want to make it that difficult for the As? Were we really that hostile, that angry? I remember how lousy I felt when America looked at the group and asked, "Will somebody please tell me what I did right? I must have done something right."

When our roles were reversed and we were the consultants, it was more of the same. The As quickly slipped into their roles as members of the nursing department, now venting their frustration and anger. As consultants we were ineffectual. Clearly it was easy to play an angry client and next to impossible to function as a helpful consultant.

"One of your problems," Mark suggested as we went over what had happened, "is that you may be comparing your skills to ours. That's not fair to yourselves. Remember we've been at this thing for a good while now; you're just in the beginning of your training."

That helped a little.

Then Irv added, "Besides, you'll never find any client as hard on you as you've been on each other."

As it turned out, he was wrong.

Toward the end of the afternoon Irv and Mark handed out our assignments for the next two weeks along with a single-spaced four-page memo on "first clients," outlining in detail the Basic Work Team intervention. Ready or not, it was going to happen.

Sitting there squeezed around that long table, I had a strong impulse to say, "Let's hold hands for a minute and say a silent prayer together."

It was one of many times in the group when I held back. I wish I hadn't. God knows we would need all the help we could get.

**Back in the Bullrushes**

The March 4 all-day session at Moses had advance billing as the day we would get ourselves together as a group—via analysis of our group climate questionnaire and, individually, via discussion of our strengths and weaknesses. This was "to insure the successful completion of the BWT intervention," according to Irv's and Mark's memo. (We never did get around to using the questionnaire into which we had put so many hours of preparation. An analysis of why the questionnaire was not used might have been helpful, but the upcoming BWT intervention had now preempted all other aspects of our training.)

As part of our homework assignment, each of us was to list, on large sheets of newsprint, his or her major strengths as well as any areas of weakness. These lists would then be used as the basis for forming consulting pairs—the next big hurdle we faced.

As I tried to work on my lists in preparation for Saturday's session, I felt a deep uneasiness. I didn't like the idea of choosing among group members, and of course I didn't know if anyone would chose to work with me. Nor did I know if I would get to do the intervention; perhaps this would turn out to be the crunch Irv had mentioned in the beginning.

The group seemed edgy and tense when we met Saturday morning. Irv greeted us with the news that Dr. F. from Harold's I & R program had left the group because of the pressure of other commitments. Dave L. was not there either; it was his wife's birthday (he never did come back to the group). We all felt let down.

Early in the session some minor incident suddenly erupted in a sharp exchange between Al W. and three of the women. As the accusations escalated, Dena S. cut in in her low, steady, yet emotional voice, "I don't think people are being honest in this group. A lot of things are going on here that nobody is talking about." In the uneasy silence that followed, I think it was America who said quietly, "I agree with Dena."

Although I didn't know specifically what Dena had referred to, I felt that Al was getting unfairly dumped on. Further, I had come to have a deep respect for Dena's observations within the group; she always seemed in touch with what was happening, particularly as it related to MLK affairs.

In this mood, we reluctantly moved to our pairing task. I think we all empathized with Gladys when she looked at Irv imploringly and said, "Can't *you* just pair us up?"

Irv's quick "No way," cut off that avenue of escape.

But once we got our lists copied on large sheets of paper and had tacked them up around the room for everyone to read, the process seemed less threatening. Now we were trying to link strengths and weaknesses rather than choosing people.

Perhaps it took 30 minutes of discussion before we came up with five consulting pairs: Ben and Gladys; Maria and Eleanor; Al and Dave; Dena and Aileen; and Valerie, Ann, and America, a triad dictated by America's exam schedule which would prevent her from taking part in the actual intervention.

I think we were all satisfied with the results except for Al being paired with Dave when he was not there. In his usual direct fashion, Al said, "I'm aware I've paid a price for the things I said earlier. But that's okay with me," he added. Al, the Leo, proud sign of the lion. Behind that pride I often felt hurt and pain. As it would work out, Al would eventually team up with Dena and me.

With the pairing out of the way, our next order of business was to start developing our entry strategy for the intervention. Irv had already given us copies of a memo he had received from Dr. A., the director of health services and as such the supervisor of the health teams, replying to Irv's long memo on the BWT intervention. Irv had already decided it should be the OD group rather than he who responded to Dr. A. The action, Irv said, was now in our hands. I think if we'd had any option we'd have given it right back to him.

The rest of that afternoon we worked up a list of thirteen contract issues to be dealt with in our meeting with Dr. A., which would be arranged as soon as possible. The preferred procedure for that meeting, we decided, was to use the "fishbowl": two or three representatives of the group would negotiate with Dr. A. while other group members observed, thus maximizing the whole group's learning.

A final session was scheduled for Tuesday evening from seven to nine in Valerie's office to take care of any further details and select our representatives to meet with Dr. A.

I don't remember any around-the-room check that afternoon before breaking, although I suppose we did one. I do remember a feeling of heaviness about the day. Outside of the prospect of working with Dena, which I looked forward to, there were none of the usual good feelings. It was as though the shadow of what was to come had already enveloped us.

### A Case of Possession?

If one were of that persuasion, a case might be made for possession as an explanation of our behavior that Tuesday night, March 7, in Valerie M.'s office. We acted that crazy. We'd had trouble before in our sessions without Irv and Mark, but never like this, never this kind of disorganization, this lack of control, this degree of frustration and anger.

Our task, at least in retrospect, should not have been that difficult. On the basis of Irv's memo on the basic work team intervention and Dr. A.'s reply, it should have been a relatively simple matter to recheck what issues remained for us to negotiate in our upcoming meeting and draft a memo to Dr. A. All that would remain would be to decide who would act as the group's representatives in the negotiations.

So why did it go so wrong? Was our anxiety and perhaps partly repressed fear of taking on this real life assignment sufficient to explain our behavior? I don't know.

I do know that anyone in the vicinity of Valerie's office that night might well have thought we were trying to recreate a scene from the Tower of Babel. Everyone seemed to be talking at once, with the decibel count constantly rising. I remember my own feelings of anger and frustration spilling over in heated exchanges. I remember counting the eight attempts Al made to say something and his being interrupted eight times. I remember Valerie standing at the board with a piece of chalk, ostensibly to list contract issues that we needed to negotiate with Dr. A., but not writing down people's suggestions. I remember Ann's question: "Valerie, do you know something the rest of us don't know?" And a little later Eleanor's repeating, "Valerie, are you *sure* you don't know something you haven't told us?"

Well, yes, as a matter of fact Valerie had already sent a memo to Dr. A. about our meeting with him.

"Sent a memo?"

"Why didn't you tell us?"

A chorus of voices.

"I guess I thought you knew I'd sent it," said Valerie matter of factly.

"How would we know?"

"Are we mind readers?"

And so on.

I remember Maria trying to calm everybody down and not succeeding very well. Then, more to assuage our feelings than anything else, it was decided a second memo should go to Dr. A. from the OD group as a whole.

When it came time to pick our representatives for Friday's meeting, everyone had reasons why he/she couldn't/wouldn't/shouldn't do it. In a final copout, we decided that Ben, who had not been able to come to this meeting, should be our spokesman. (As Irv would later point out, we felt we *had* to have a doctor to represent us with Dr. A. and Ben was the only remaining MD in the group.) If Ben would do it, Eleanor would also take on the assignment. Maria, it was decided, would act as facilitator—although I don't think we were ever clear on the why or how of her role. Anything to get finished and out of that room.

There was a special bonus for our performance that night. Dr. A., whose office was two down from Valerie's, was also working late. He could not have failed to be aware of the tenor of what was happening in the OD group meeting so close by.

That Friday morning at 9 we met Dr. A. in one of the classrooms at the center generally used for training purposes. Ben, Eleanor, and Maria sat at a largish table in the center of the room, the rest of us in chairs against the wall. Dr. A. was a few minutes late in arriving, and when he came he was obviously irritated.

Dr. A. was one of the first superstars in the social medicine internship and residency program at Montefiore; he had moved from I&R into his present post of director of health services at the MLK Center. A double Aries with Scorpio rising, he was a powerhouse of drive and energy. He worked incredibly hard and expected the same of others. Besides his medical training, he had worked with the late community activist Saul Alinsky on community development projects and was a staunch advocate of moving community people into all top management positions in the center. He also had read extensively in management literature and considered himself a proponent of Theory Y—although his style and directiveness often made him come across more X than Y.[2]

In the next 35 minutes Dr. A. would give one of his virtuoso performances. Ben, whose greatest difficulty in the group had been in confronting conflict, was no match for him that morning. Nor was Eleanor. Nor would any of us have been.

After stating that he didn't like to have his time wasted and that most of the issues raised in our second memo had already been covered in his memo to Irv, he went into action. Did we consider ourselves an operational group? Dr. A. wanted to know.

"Operational? Why, yes, we're operational," Ben answered.

"In that case," Dr. A. said, "I will expect all of you, as part of my line organization, to report to me everything that happens in your work with the teams. You will name names, you will spell out specific incidents, you will keep me informed at all times on everyone with whom you have contact."

Glazed looks. Low murmurs from the back row.

Dr. A.'s sharp "You said you were operational, didn't you?"

And so it went for 30 minutes.

Toward the end Dr. A. relented. We were not, of course, he explained, operational or part of his line organization. And, of course, he didn't expect us to name names, etc. A general report on our team interventions and the viability of the BWT concept was what he wanted from us. Now, since he was very busy, and since there were no more questions, he'd be leaving. With that he went out the door.

We sat there in stunned silence. Negotiating a contract with Dr. A. was something else!

**The Ides Plus One**

Irv had already gotten the word on what had happened before he met with the group in the long narrow room in the Community Health Advocacy offices on East 169th Street late in the afternoon of March 16. Mark was not with him that day; we could have used his quiet, helpful comments. As we found places around the long table, I thought I had never seen Irv look so grim. Well, he could hardly be pleased with the performance of his trainees.

Irv was starting to talk. There were certain things, he said, that we needed to seriously consider as the group's work was coming to an end.

An end? Nobody had said anything about an end before. We were a learning group and this was our first intervention. What end?

Not everyone, Irv went on, is cut out for OD or the facilitator role. Some of us might find this to be the case. And with our work as a group drawing to a close *(there it was again),* it would be well to recognize this.

It was Gladys who finally spoke up, "I thought we were in training, that we were going to be an OD department. I feel we've just started. How can this group end?"

Well, Irv said, this phase of the training is winding up with the BWT intervention. Then it will be up to each one of you to decide where you want to go. An OD department, he added, is not necessarily the best strategy.

*What was going on?* I looked at Valerie. She was staring impassively at the table. Something *had* happened. But it would be several weeks before I knew that indeed a decision had been made to drop the idea of an OD department and that the future of this group was in fact very much up in the air. That March evening, I think most of us felt we were being punished for having blown our first contract setting assignment, that Irv just didn't believe we were good enough.

As we sat silently trying to comprehend what was happening, Irv changed pace. That afternoon, he said, he had received from Dr. A. a list of five basic work team units, each made up of an internist, pediatrician, nurse, and family health worker. Dr. A. had selected these groups because they functioned well and would probably be receptive to the experiment we planned. Each consulting pair could now decide which unit it wanted to work with. It was a relief to turn to a specific task, and with a kind of glum determination we got on with the job.

The procedure we were to follow seemed simple enough. Each pair was to contact Dr. A's secretary within the next day or two to set up an appointment for the following week if possible, at which time Dr. A. would introduce the OD pair to the team and briefly explain the purpose of the basic work team intervention. Then he would bow out and the two OD people could answer any questions and explain how they would work.

The game plan we were to follow was in many ways like a condensed version of the work MIT had done with the large teams. After an initial contract setting session—which would deal with what we needed from the BWT members and what they could expect to get from us—we would interview each member individually.

After we had pooled the data from the interviews and organized it around key issues, we would meet with the four-member unit for a feedback session. This, in essence, would be like saying, "Okay, here is your data. Now what do you want to do about it?" This would then lead to the action planning phase.

Our primary concern was to be the group's goals and roles; we were told not to expect to tackle any heavy interpersonal issues. The whole intervention was to take no more than ten to twelve hours and would involve three or four sessions with the basic work team members.

On the way home that night, I thought, "It's good we have something concrete to work on." I tried to push the other things that had happened out of my mind.

### Introductions

As it worked out, Dena and I were the first pair to get launched. We were to meet Dr. A. in the team's office at 8:45 Monday morning. The team secretary was supposed to have informed all team members of the meeting. She had—except for the doctors. "Doctors," said Dr. A. tartly, "are also members of MLK health teams."

Despite some delay in rounding up missing members, fifteen or twenty minutes later we were all seated in Room 408. Dr. A. spoke briefly of OD and the basic work team concept. He emphasized his concern for finding ways to improve the delivery of health care to patients. Hopefully this experiment, he said, would help in achieving this objective. Of course, he continued, this was a voluntary activity, "but if any of the four BWT members I've designated decides not to participate, she had better have an excellent reason."

Because of the delay in starting, when Dr. A. had finished his brief presentation our time had run out. No questions, no discussion were possible. All we got was an agreement to meet with the four BWT members early in the week to work out the ground rules, to set the contract under which we would operate.

### Mini Intervention

Irv and Mark had both stressed that this was a mini intervention. As they put it in one of their memos to us, "In no way are you to think of this as a magnum opus on health team functioning."

I do not think any of us did. But what we quickly discovered was that even a mini intervention required a surprising number of hours just to plan for our work sessions with the BWT. The OD group's last full day together at Moses on Saturday, March 25, was entirely devoted to such planning.

During the morning we went over data collection issues in terms of the individual interviews we would be conducting with BWT members. Then we moved on to data summary issues, issues concerning the managing of the feedback-action planning sessions, and issues around how we would work together as a consulting pair. We spent time examining dimensions of our objectives: We were to focus on task related issues; that is, "How can the BWT improve the health care it delivers to a given family?" We talked about our role in helping to legitimize and formalize what was now, at best, an informal system. We looked at what work needs to get done to improve the management/coordination of total care for a patient population. And we went over the key role of the family health worker as central contact for client families.

As the day progressed I felt more and more as though I was trying to memorize dozens of rules which I had to keep repeating inside my head or they'd all disappear. (In fact, it wasn't until they had disappeared—at least from my head—that I was able to function effectively.)

In the afternoon, when we broke into pairs to do an analysis of the factors working for and against the BWT concept at the MLK Center, Al joined Dena and me and we became a working trio. As such we would meet our four-person group the following Tuesday to set the contract that would govern our work together.

That night as I tried to sort out and sift through the many guidelines we had been given, I could not dismiss the feeling that there was some confusion in the OD people's role in this intervention. Were we BWT advocates, attempting to sell the concept to the teams? Or was our role to be primarily facilitative, to help BWT members determine for themselves whether this organizational change would help them to improve the delivery of patient care? Sometimes it sounded like one, sometimes like the other.

**Setting the Contract**

Dena, Al, and I met on Tuesday to go over our schedule once more before the session started. As our BWT members drifted into Room 402, we tried to appear relaxed. After all, this was only a mini intervention.

We had a few extra minutes before the session formally started while we waited for the internist, who was on her way back to MLK from a teaching assignment at Montefiore. The pediatrician, a warm, voluble, dominant woman, spoke at some length about how well this group worked together, how well they got along together. There were nodding assents from the nurse and family health worker.

When the internist arrived, we started by once again going over the BWT concept: "The basic work team is defined by a group of about 150 families, whose health care is 'managed' by one family health worker, who is assisted by a public health nurse, an internist, and a pediatrician, as well as other support people who provide services as needed."

"Any questions?"

Silence.

Then we spelled out the goal of this experiment: We were going to try to determine whether formalizing and extending the BWT throughout all the health teams would serve to improve the quality and quantity of health care provided.

"Any questions?"

Silence.

To answer this basic question, we would need to interview each group member individually. Then, after we had pooled the data from all the interviews, we would meet again as a group to diagnose the problems and develop some action plans, based on the data they had given us.

As I watched the faces of our BWT members while we talked of goals and roles, the feeling I got was one of passive resistance. These people were here because they had been told to be here, but their expectations of anything useful to them coming out of this experiment, I suspected, were minimal.

When we again asked if there were questions or comments, the pediatrician started talking. Since there were no problems within their group, she said she really didn't understand why they had been selected for this experiment. Why not select some of the people who were having problems?

The idea, we replied, was to pick well-functioning groups so we could all better understand how they worked together to get the job done.

"I don't belong in this group anyway," the nurse said. "I only share about fifteen of the family health worker's families. Mrs. X (the other nurse on the team) should be here, not me."

Did she want to speak to Dr. A. about this since he had selected the group? Her answer was a shrug. It didn't make that much difference, she seemed to say.

When the session was over, Dena, Al, and I reviewed what had happened. Under the circumstances, it probably had gone as well as could be expected. Anyway, we'd made a start. And as part of our "contract," we had agreed to meet again as a group on April 17, which would give us a little more than two weeks to collect the data and organize it for the first feedback session.

**Collecting the Data**

Our interviews were to be structured around four key questions:

1. What kinds of tasks and problems would require the four members to meet together? (What, when, where, why?)
2. What responsibilities must *each* member assume if the basic work team is to operate most effectively?
3. What are the barriers to such functioning (such as time constraints or space constraints)?

4. What environmental changes may be necessary for BWTs to function effectively?

Irv and Mark had suggested half an hour as an appropriate amount of time for each interview. We found it took much longer. Sticking to the questions as outlined was difficult. And, unlike the group session, in individual interviews people were eager to talk and had a lot to say, some of which did not readily fit within our defined format. In one instance a second interview had to be scheduled.

Later, as Dena, Al, and I tried to integrate the data we had collected, it was clear that formalizing the basic work team concept did not provoke great enthusiasm, although the nurse provided some support. Increased patient loads, longer hours of work, the many recent organizational changes at MLK had produced a kind of weariness as well as a skepticism toward experimenting with any further changes.

Everyone spoke of time constraints, particularly the internist and pediatrician, who would be the common denominator in six basic work teams. "I can't get everything done now, so how can I possibly be expected to meet regularly with six different groups of people? Besides that," the pediatrician had said, "the BWT concept just won't work with some of the people on the team. It's better to leave things as they are than try to change them." She did agree that communication on a one-to-one basis was often not adequate when it came to the multiple-problem family (an adult with TB, a battered child, and a teenager on drugs all in one household). Even with TB alone, she allowed, a coordinated approach to the whole family's health care, involving the family health worker, public health nurse, internist, and pediatrician, would be far more effective than the present piecemeal method of dealing with such problems. "But we have no time for this kind of planning, and it's unrealistic to expect it with the patient loads we carry. We're doing the very best we can now."

The internist saw it a bit differently. "The real problem," she said in her interview, "is to bring on board team members who feel they are outsiders and help them to work more effectively. This would have a payoff for the whole team as well as for the families we care for."

"Would the BWT help achieve this?"

"I'm not sure," was her reply. "Perhaps an informal network of BWTs could help, and if so I'd support it. Of course, each family health worker should be linked with a nurse, a pediatrician, and an internist for each of her families; and the nurses and doctors should recognize their responsibilities to assist the family health workers. As it is now, some people don't know where to go to get assistance."

Then she added, "But I'd be concerned if the BWT weakened the larger team. With all our problems, we've still come a long way since our work with MIT. I think I could only support the BWT concept if it complemented and enhanced the larger team's functioning."

The family health worker appeared skeptical, perhaps ambivalent, then fatalistic. "If they've decided 'upstairs' that they're going to have BWTs," she said, averting her eyes, "I don't think it's going to make a bit of difference how we feel about it down here. We certainly have problems on our team, but I don't know if this BWT thing is an answer; I don't know if it would help or just take up more time. I think we need more of the MIT kind of help. That really made a difference."

"Would you be willing to experiment with the BWT on the larger team to see if it would work?"

"I might be willing to experiment," she said, then added, "if the others wanted to."

The strongest support for the BWT came from the nurse, who felt this might be a way to provide better family health care through better planning and coordination. "So much of what we do now is on a crisis basis. I'd like to get away from that as much as possible," she added.

Also, since she herself had experienced difficulty when she first came on the team, she saw the BWT as a possible vehicle for more successfully linking the various providers of health care services. "If I had been assigned to a BWT unit when I first came on the team, I think it could have speeded up my being accepted as a functioning health team member. As it was, I was just kind of ignored. It made me feel bad."

These were just some of the pertinent pieces of information Dena, Al, and I had gathered in the course of our interviewing. But the wealth of material, we soon recognized, presented its own brand of headache. How to condense it, how to organize it? These were problems we faced.

After two long, exhausting sessions lasting well into the evening, we managed to reduce the material to a page and a half (single spaced, typewritten) of data feedback. The agenda we worked out for the coming session was simple: after discussing the objectives of the meeting and briefly restating our contract with the group, we would focus on "working" the data and end up with a summary of where we'd been and what would come next.

But it didn't turn out quite that way.

### Data Feedback

I think we got through discussing the objectives of the meeting and I know we handed out copies of the data feedback sheets, but no one really looked at them. Instead we were quickly inundated with a wave of invective about other team members (no one here, of course) who didn't carry their weight, who were impossible to work with, who should be fired, who never cooperated. No BWT, it was emphasized, could ever work with such people. And so on.

Attempts by Dena, by Al, by me to get the focus back within the group, back on their own data, were met with a frontal attack on us. We were there to push the BWT; we didn't care what they had to say. The outcome of this experiment, they suggested, had been decided before it ever started.

Whatever tentative support had previously existed for the BWT had now evaporated. Our only accomplishment in that 1½ hour session was to get their agreement to go over the data summary before our next session on May 2, which was the earliest date they could all meet with us again.

Nor did our next OD group session shortly after help very much. Dena was not there and when our data summary came under attack from the group—it was unfocused, too long, not clear, tried to cover too much—Al quickly disassociated himself from it (he had had to leave that planning session early—but Al, how could you desert me now?). I felt as though I was the target in a shooting gallery. When Irv looked at me and said, "You'd better get some help before your next session," the way I heard it it might as well have been, "You better turn yourself in to Bellevue Psychiatric for treatment." Valerie, who was sitting next to me, said in a lowered voice, "It's hard to look good in this group no matter what you do." I silently assented.

That night, after a long phone conversation with Dena, I did what I had done many times before during the OD training. I searched through our reading assignments, looking for some insight into, some understanding of, what had happened.

The article on planned change seemed particularly relevant. Well into it, I came to the sentence *"No matter what the changes are, there is likely to be some resistance to change."* And, a couple of sentences further, *"If an organization tried every new scheme, product, or process that came along it would soon wander aimlessly, flounder, and die. The positive function of resistance to change is to insure that plans for change and their ultimate consequences are thought through carefully."* And then, *"Another cause of resistance to change can be the sudden imposition of changes in someone's environment without that person's prior knowledge of, or participation in, that change."*

As I underscored these words, I wondered if the BWT members perceived us as coming to them with solutions to problems rather than providing some problem solving skills that they themselves could use. I thought of the family health worker's words: "If they've decided upstairs that they're going to have BWTs, I don't think it makes a bit of difference how we feel about it down here."

Perhaps in our desire to do a good job we had been pushing a solution—the BWT. If so, of course we had met resistance and resentment. In fact, we had created them ourselves!

I thought back to our Enterprise-Merger exercise with the paper airplanes; of how angry we Enterprise people had been when our Merger "consultants" seemed to be pushing solutions at us. And what could possibly be gained by forcing a "solution" anyway? Hadn't we found out, in our first day of training at Moses, that there was literally no commitment to implement a decision that one didn't really support?

All these thoughts were reassuring to me. I remembered Mark's saying early in our training that nobody really wins or loses in these exercises, but hopefully everybody learns. Maybe we had already learned something important in our mini intervention. I'd have to check it with Dena and Al.

### Stress Facilitator Role

When the three of us met a few days later we asked Ben to sit in with us as a process observer. Ben was very good in this role and helped us clarify some of our problems. I wondered now why Irv's suggestion that we better get some help had seemed so ominous to me only a few days ago. Getting and giving help, after all, was what this training was about. Yet most of us, I recognized, were still reluctant to admit we needed assistance from each other—or, more importantly, that we could get assistance from one another. Not yet trusting ourselves in the OD role, neither could we trust other group members.

As we went over with Ben what had happened in the last BWT session, we decided to emphasize the facilitator role; we were there to assist BWT members to define their problems and examine possible solutions. If they decided to experiment further with the BWT concept, very good. If they decided on some other course of action, that was okay too.

We also decided to redo the data in simpler form, grouping key statements under three major headings. Our plan for the May 2 session was to briefly review our contract with BWT members, stressing their agreement to work on their own data and, with our assistance, develop some action plans around the problems they had identified. It sounded okay; now we'd have to see if it worked.

The amazing thing to the three of us was how well the May 2 meeting went. Clarifying our OD role had lessened the tension we experienced. And perhaps their ventilation in the previous session had helped clear the air a bit for them. Whatever the reason, they now seemed ready to deal with the problems they had identified. Also we noticed that a subtle shift had taken place within the group. Initially dominated by the pediatrician, the other three members, with encouragement from us, were now more willing to speak up, to make suggestions, to take initiative. Our original contract had provided for only two feedback-planning sessions. They suggested another meeting and also asked Dena to sit in on their next full team meeting to make a brief presentation on the BWT.

We were all delighted.

As I thought about it that evening, I realized that the feeling of having to remember dozens of rules had disappeared some time during today's session. Things were starting to fall into place—many pieces finally forming a meaningful whole, an intelligent pattern. All the failures, confusions, frustrations I'd experienced so often during the training now seemed justified. I felt a warmth toward the whole group, toward Irv and Mark, the BWT people we worked with, and most of all toward my colleagues Dena and Al.

**Saying Goodbye**

During the weeks of our involvement in the BWT experiment, the larger group had receded in importance. Each pair or triad was so absorbed in the work it was doing that we had only the haziest idea where the other groups were. When we did meet with Irv and Mark, it was mostly to go over what had happened with the consulting pairs and plan the next steps.

But now, as we were coming to the end of the intervention, the larger group once again assumed central importance. The intervention experience, difficult as it was at times, had given all of us a confidence we had lacked before; a confidence to start trusting ourselves and to start trusting each other.

Our task now was the preparation of our reports on the BWT experiment. On May 17 Irv and Mark met with us to work out a general format for these reports. That morning, coming uptown on the rickety old Third Avenue El, I thought: Spring has even come to the South Bronx. The tinned-over windows in gutted buildings which stared vacantly as the El train, like some giant caterpillar, wound its way north did not seem as depressing as they had on so many other occasions.

When I arrived at the CHA offices where we were meeting that day, I could hear birds calling in the bushes outside the window. As people came in with their sandwich lunches, I checked around the circle. We numbered eleven, including Irv and Mark. Six of the eleven, I counted, were born in the sign of Gemini (no other sign was represented by more than one person).

"Hey," I said, "we should have a party to celebrate all the Gemini birthdays."

We didn't, of course, but the feeling of celebration was real: We had come through the initiating fire; we had survived.

Before the first week in June the four BWT reports had been completed and, with a covering section by Irv and Mark that reviewed the larger implications of the experiment, had been sent along to MLK's top management.

Our contract was now completed. We were at the end. Valeria, Maria, and Al would go to Bethel in July for two weeks of laboratory training in human relations. While other members' schedules did not permit that much time away at present, shorter training labs might be possible later on. There were always training opportunities if one was determined.

The group? Would we meet again? Would we continue? It was up to us, Irv and Mark had insisted; the initiative was in our hands.

I don't think any of us believed that without the specific backing of MLK's top management, without a specific objective for our coming together, that we would make it on our own. We hadn't come that far; we weren't that sure. Other pressures would prevail.

"I don't know when I'll see you again," said Ann when I ran into her on the street near the center a couple of weeks later.

"We must get the group together soon," I answered. But it was more wish than plan of action. I was an outsider again. Our paths were going in separate directions.

## PART III—ADDING IT UP

As a different kind of outsider—one who looks through whatever is the opposite of rose colored glasses—it would be easy to assume that the OD intervention training was something of a bust at MLK. Like the concept of the basic work team, organization development might seem to be an idea whose time has not yet arrived. No further training with the MIT people has been scheduled for either middle managers or a new group of OD intervenors. And one will look in vain in the 1972 MLK annual report for any mention of this program that started with so much riding on it, with such high expectations for its success.

Was the OD training the failure this might suggest?

Before calling for any requiems, the intervention training should be viewed in terms of at least two factors: (1) the results of the trainees' work with the BWTs, and (2) what the OD-trained people have done in the agency in the eight months since their training ended.

The basic work team reports are perhaps the most clear-cut evidence of the OD training program's success. All four reports are proof of the trainees' ability to carry out what in fact was not an easy assignment. Ben and Gladys, who avoided the advocate role from the beginning, were probably most effective as facilitators, providing their group with problem solving skills that members could then make use of on their own. For the rest of us, the more closely we identified with the BWT advocacy role the more difficulty we had in the intervention. Yet despite the role ambiguity that most of us experienced, we were all able to complete the assignment and to independently reach the conclusion that formalization of the basic work team would not be useful in achieving improved patient care—at least not at that time. In all the reports, further experimentation with the BWT was recommended, preferably involving a whole team next time around. The usefulness of this organizational arrangement could thus be tested as it would actually operate if it were put into effect. This would also provide a vehicle for dealing with some of the more pressing problems identified by BWT members, such as breakdowns in communication, uneven work loads, role confusion (most members were not sure what they needed to get from other members to get their work done or what others needed to get from them to function more effectively), and so on.

On the basis of these reports I think the training rates high marks. The fact that no further experimentation was done to test the possible usefulness of the BWT structure was a management decision that does not reflect on the competence of the OD trainees. (See Appendices A and B to this chapter for Irv's and Mark's evaluation of the OD training program at the time it was completed and their overview of the BWT interventions.)

Another way of evaluating the training program is to look at the job performance of the people who participated in it. All of them, without exception, say they have been able to utilize the intervention skills they learned in training, and most of them feel this has enhanced the quality and the quantity of their work at MLK.

Eleanor M., who is now deputy director of health services and as such a member of the top management group, is in possibly the toughest job in the agency (as supervisor of the medical staff, she has direct contact with physicians and nurses, some of whom are not overly enthusiastic about community control, particularly if it means reporting to a nonmedically trained female person). She obviously needs and she makes use of her OD skills in working with groups and individuals.

Dena S. has gone on to larger responsibilities in setting up a drug addiction program and working closely with the schools in the area on drug related problems. Gladys V. and America C. are unit managers, each responsible for supervising two health teams. Ann S. continues her work as public health nurse and uses her OD skills on the health team as well as with the patients she sees. Al W. was faced with a critical decision regarding his career and more importantly his life: he decided against taking a top management position, which would require an investment in time and energy he decided should go instead to his family and his church work.

Maria R. and Ben S. have both left the agency, Ben to work in the Boston area on health teams using his OD experience; Maria to take on new training responsibilities at Montefiore.

### From Valerie's Vantage

What about Valerie M., chairman of the OD effort and key person in our group? Shortly after our training program ended, Valerie talked at some length with me about the experience and what it had meant to her. Because of the importance of her perceptions, both to MLK and to an understanding of many of the things that happened in our training program, I want to quote extensively from the transcribed tape of that interview.

> I had a lot of problems with the group from the beginning. First, I didn't really want to be in it. But Irv and Bill Lloyd kind of pushed me. So I said, okay, I'd do it. But there were times when I came very close to dropping out.
>
> It started off badly for me when the first thing the MLK people wanted to know was whether anyone would drive them over to Moses. Now that would have been the last thing I would have thought of. I'd assume that it was my responsibility to get myself wherever I was supposed to be. It really made me mad, but I couldn't talk about it in the group. I guess I didn't have that much trust at the time.
>
> Another thing: I wanted the group to be perfect. When I had to recognize that the group wasn't perfect—that not all of the twelve

people who had been selected for the training were going to make it—I had to do a lot of work trying to understand how my high expectations affect others as well as myself. I always have high expectations; I make very heavy demands. But I've had to face it that not everybody is going to get things done as quickly as I want them to.

Another thing I have with groups: I tend to go to one of two extremes; either I take over or I don't get involved at all. It's hard for me to hit a happy medium. To feel really comfortable, I have to have a little more knowledge, a little more data than anybody else.

The thing is I have to look good. I can't stand being seen as a failure. Now add to that the fact that not only was I a member of the group, but according to the agency, the OD group was my responsibility. As chairman of the group, I felt everyone expected me to be some kind of expert on OD, to really know what it was all about. But I wasn't an expert; I didn't know any more about OD than the others. Still, I didn't want them to know that I didn't kno which put me in an awful bind. I just kind of receded, didn't partic pate, didn't say much. It was about this time that Irv said to me, "You don't learn when you're not involved. You're not investing anything." But I didn't feel like I wanted to invest anything then.

It wasn't until I got a sense of knowing what it was all about that I felt I could open up in the group. What I didn't realize in the begi ning was that this created a problem for the group. I just saw it as problem. It was a long time before I realized that group members were really concerned about me. I didn't see it at first.

This is connected with the whole problem of getting help. There are times when I want people to help me (I need their help to get n work done). But I don't know how to ask for help. And then I get angry when people don't give me help. I think a lot of people arou the agency are like that—a lot of us have difficulty asking for help. It's too much like being dependent or saying you can't do the job c your own. I think it's one of the reasons I had such a hard time in the blindfold exercise. I was petrified when Maria was supposed to take me across Gun Hill Road; I could hear the traffic; I was sure I was going to get hit; and Maria would just keep on talking. I nearly pulled the blindfold off I was so scared. The whole exercise was scary, but I think I learned a lot from it. It's pretty uncomfortable to be helpless—that's one thing. The other thing is that you have to trust some people some times; there's no other way.

Another thing about this training: I'm very impatient with what I call the noncontent thing—you know, I hear a lot of words but I don't see specific things that I can latch onto and use right away. So when we spend time in the group on process, I get impatient, maybe turn off, because I don't see the relevance.

I thought in this training that I would learn some skills. Then I'd be able to apply them. And that would be that—period. After a wh

> I began to realize that in order to be able to practice these skills, OD has to become almost a part of the person, that in certain ways the person is going to have to change. That's something I didn't bargain for; I didn't think I needed changing that much. But as it turned out, it helped me in my work here and with my family at home.
>
> I'm still very work-oriented, but I think I'm learning to be a little more patient. I've begun to look at people a little differently. Before, I'd make an evaluation very quickly; if the person didn't meet my standards, that was it. Then I began to see that by this kind of snap-judgment elimination, I had a very small pool of people to draw on. And that even if the person didn't have every quality I was looking for, he or she could still make important contributions. This has really helped me and I'm doing it much more often.
>
> So while I didn't get what I expected from the training, maybe it will turn out that I got something even more important. I don't know; I guess it will take time to find out.

There is little doubt that everyone in the group benefited from the OD training program. Yet the question has to be asked: Why hasn't MLK made use of the trainees' skills in an organized way in the center? Why hasn't the program been continued?

**Management's Problem**

Part of the answer no doubt lies in one of the points Irv and Mark made in their review of the training: MLK management did not sufficiently understand organization development and what is required to implement OD concepts; it didn't really know *how* to make use of the OD capability once it had been developed.

Parenthetically, considering the problems we had as trainees in making connections between our experiential exercises and becoming sufficiently skillful to take on the BWT intervention, it should surprise no one that people who have not gone through the training would find it difficult to see how the agency could use the trainees' new skills other than in the jobs they are doing.

There is another factor that may in part account for the failure to build on this program: the long range goal of developing an internal OD capability that would play a key role in helping the agency become a self-renewing organization somehow got submerged in the BWT intervention. Originally seen as simply providing an initial field experience for the trainees, the BWT experiment became almost an end in itself. When the decision was made to drop the BWT, for many it was synonomous with dropping the OD training. Somehow the two concepts had become intertwined; if one went under, so did the other.

This also relates to the trainees' own role confusion in the intervention. If our job was to persuade the teams to adopt the BWT structure, then indeed we failed. But if we were involved as facilitators in an experiment to see if the structure should be extended, then there was no failure. In this respect, the expectations of management and the expectations of our trainers may have been very different.

The problem of expectations was further elaborated by Valerie in the taped interview. What she expected to learn, she said, were some skills, which she would then be able to apply in her job. That's a very long distance, as she reports, from recognizing that one must be open to changing oneself, that OD is a great deal more than a series of skills or a bag of tricks. The feelings involved in any such recognition can range from unsettling to something close to terrifying.

Finally, add to this the picture of a health center everlastingly swamped in impossible tasks; a health center in the process of bringing community people into all managerial jobs, from unit managers to project director; a health center whose funding is in gravest jeopardy with OEO's imminent demise. Given these realities, it takes little imagination to see the handwriting on the wall.

And yet, despite all these and many other problems, the "fit" between the center's objectives and OD is too good to give up on. Briefly, consider just one of MLK's original goals: to involve families in taking responsibility for their own health care. If this goal is ever to be achieved, it seems likely that the providers of health services will need to demonstrate not only care and concern for their patients (clients) but also self-reliance, initiative, responsibility—the qualities they want to help instill in their families.

Such qualities are not fostered in an organization run by edict by a small group at the top. Again quoting from the article on planned change:

> The process of growth and maturation is one of gaining mastery over one's environment. Management by imposed change serves to arrest this process by denying subordinates the opportunity to live in an environment they can understand and control. Men who spend their lives in organizations managed by imposed change can become helpless, passive victims of the system, cursed by management for their stupidity and lack of initiative.

The center simply cannot afford to have employees—at any level—who lack initiative or who behave stupidly.

In contrast to top-down management, organization development provides the tools for building a structure that encourages people to become self-actualizing, to take risks, to assume responsibilities.

The kind of commitment, dedication, and intelligence that the trainees brought to the OD training program—at the same time they carried on incredibly demanding full-time jobs—is an asset MLK might well make better use of in working toward the goal of creating a self-renewing organization with its own internal OD capability.

And perhaps it will happen. After a period of germination, spring must surely come again to the South Bronx.

## NOTES

1. Matthew B. Miles, *Learning to Work in Groups* (New York: Teachers College Press, Columbia University, 1959). This and E.H. Schein's *Process Consultation* (Reading, Mass.: Addison-Wesley, 1969) were our two basic texts, supplemented with material from various other sources.
2. Douglas McGregor, in his now classic *New Patterns of Management* (New York: McGraw-Hill, 1960), formulated the Theory X, Theory Y concept of managing. Very briefly, he believed that Theory Y managers operate on the assumption that people do not inherently dislike work but rather, under proper conditions, seek responsibility and want to perform effectively. It is the manager's job to create the conditions that will encourage people to so function. The Theory X manager, on the other hand, assumes that people are generally lazy, dislike work and responsibility, and can only be motivated by extrinsic rewards and punishment. He manages on the basis of these assumptions.

# Appendix A

*TO:* *MLK Top Management*
*FROM:* *Irv Rubin and Mark Plovnick*
*SUBJECT:* *Evaluation of OD Training* *Date:* *June 21, 1972*

### History

The idea of having an internal OD capability had been discussed for many months. It wasn't until MLK began to get a sense of what OD really was (and was not) that this abstract idea became operationally feasible. The need to do some experimental work with the basic work team concept provided the necessary stimulus and point of focus around which to consider an institutional investment in developing an internal OD capability.

### Goals

A training program was begun to develop a cadre of people from within MLK with basic OD skills. This group's first field experience would involve their working with selected basic work team units, but their raison d'être was not limited to this initial intervention. Rather, among other specific objectives, the BWT intervention was to be a stepping stone and developmental opportunity. Ultimately we hoped to have a group of internal OD resources able to intervene and facilitate in team development and other activities at MLK and perhaps in other centers as well.

### Evaluation of the OD Training Program

Based on our own observations of the participants in the OD training and on their reported experiences in the BWT intervention, we would evaluate the training a success. That is, the center now has a number of resources that can be called upon to facilitate certain activities involving team development and other change efforts, and who can enhance their skills and the scope of their activities by pursuing any of a number of different educational opportunities that are available to them. These include further exposure to MIT training, courses at local universities, and training experiences available through the National Training Laboratories and other OD training organizations.

In this report we will describe some of the factors contributing to the success of the OD training program we developed with this group, as well as those factors which seemed to impede the group's progress. This analysis is based on evaluations done by each individual participant in the training program as well as by ourselves. The results presented here are organized into factors concerning (1) the consultants, (2) the participants, and (3) other people at the center and the general environment. It should be noted, and will be discussed in our conclusions, that factors listed in any one category have implications for the other categories. This is important if we are to draw on our experience to improve future training programs.

### Consultants—Positive Factors

1. Irv and Mark have "complementary" styles and skills.
2. Irv and Mark share a strong desire to see both MLK and OD at MLK succeed.
3. Irv and Mark represent a wide variety of experiences, particularly in training change agents in other settings, which were brought to bear in this effort.

### Consultants—Negative Factors

1. Our strong desires for this group's success led to our overpushing and setting a very fast pace. In retrospect, we tried to do a tremendous amount with a novice group, all of whom held *full-time jobs,* in a very short period of time. A colleague summed it up with the question, "What's the hurry?" Actually the 80-odd hours we will have spent with this group is "equivalent" to a year's course work at MIT. For this pace we have traded off several things:
   A. The pace—our's and MLK's—eliminated much opportunity for the trainee's personal reflection and individual integration of "what this means to me as a potential OD person."
   B. Except within actual training sessions, only limited opportunity was available for peer group learning via interaction.
   C. The pace did not allow much time for conceptual understanding and therefore tended to deemphasize this part of the learning experience.
2. Coupled with the pace has been a very directive style on our part. We have pushed hard and tried to absorb and deal with the group's natural anxiety as functionally as possible. This made the group quite dependent on us, though the confidence they gained from their BWT intervention helped alleviate this situation.
3. During the course of the training we did not keep top management sufficient-

ly informed of our progress and problems. Thus management's expectations for the OD group were and are unclear to top management, to us, and to OD group members themselves. This confusion raises doubts in the center as to the role of internal OD resources and about management's commitment to OD activities.

4. We tended to accept certain strategy decisions made by ourselves and others without considering their implications for our overall success. For example, the criteria used by management to select participants, in retrospect, raised some questions. Particularly interesting was the criterion that the group be "representative of the agency." The immediate strength of this approach, from our point of view, was the fact that the OD group would consequently be a microcosm of the center. As a "learning organization" we would experience many of the same dilemmas as other interdisciplinary groups at MLK. The resulting learning potential was attractive.

   It is unclear to us whether a very different group would have been selected if this criterion had not been applied. From our point of view, the group we have is a good one—motivated, committed, and generally capable of grasping important material quickly. We are also aware, however, that community-based systems can overemphasize representation, possibly at the expense of achievement. This is a point we will have to rethink carefully when new groups are considered.

   Other examples of accepting strategies too readily include the design of the basic work team experiment, which we describe in the BWT report [see Appendix B to this chapter], and the departmental status we initially accepted as the ultimate destiny of the OD group. With respect to the latter, there is evidence from industry, and other organizations that maintain formal OD departments, that this arrangement often places OD department members in a very vulnerable position in times of organization stress, and reduces the level of risk they can assume in the conduct of their OD activities. A more integrated distribution of OD resources—i.e., not a formal department—has generally been more effective.

#### Participants—Positive Factors

1. Prior experience of some group members with OD in the initial MIT team intervention.
2. Experience on MLK teams enhancing their knowledge of team and center problems.
3. High commitments to the center's goals and values.
4. Willingness to work hard to learn OD skills—partly as a result of a desire to expand career opportunities.
5. Diversity of abilities and orientation in the group made them a "microcosm" of the center.

### Participants—Negative Factors

1. Commitment varied. Some members dropped out or were unable to devote as much time and energy as was necessary to develop OD skills.
2. Even as we were doing role-playing simulations, the role problems this OD group faces became obvious. They have a content-process dilemma. Each is a content expert in an area of health care. The tendency to overemphasize those content skills vs. their newly learned OD skills will be strong for two reasons: (a) the role expectations their clients have of them; and (b) their own, hopefully short-lived, anxiety about their skills as OD people.
3. There was a general hesitancy among group members to confront each other, or us, around various issues that were important to their training. This low-risk tendency can probably be attributed in part to the low-risk, nonexperimental climate found at the center in general, as well as to personal characteristics of the OD group participants, and to our training strategies (e.g., our directive style).

### Other People and the Environment—Positive Factors

1. The training program could never have started without the commitment of Harold Wise to MLK, and the commitment of the center's top management to having an OD capability.
2. As MLK is seen as the "model experiment" by people outside the center, activities such as this experimental training program are encouraged through availability of funding, and through contagious enthusiasm.

### Other People and the Environment—Negative Factors

1. Outside funding *may* reduce the level of active OD involvement of the center's management below that which might occur if the program was being paid for by the center.
2. A lack of understanding by the center concerning the time involved in learning OD skills often led to difficulty for participants in securing free time for training sessions.
3. Time problems are of course compounded by the hectic pace of work throughout the center.
4. Accommodations that are appropriate—i.e., quiet, comfortable, and nearby—for the kind of training involved are hard to come by at the center.

### Conclusions

In analyzing a change strategy, it is generally more effective to reduce negative or restraining factors than to increase positive or helping factors. Increasing positive forces often leads to a generally higher level of tension in a system (negative forces usually increase or develop to meet positive forces), while decreasing the negative factors generally reduces tension and leads to longer term change. Thus, in planning for a next round of training it is most appropriate to concentrate on ways to reduce the negative forces identified in our analysis.

One of the most pervasive factors with negative impact was the perceived sense of urgency that led to the high pressure pace of training. Partly this reflects our own expectations, but to a large extent it reflects the nature of activity at the center in general. The center's pace became our pace and was reinforced by center concerns over the amount of time being devoted to OD by the participants. We all need to recognize that to train OD resources effectively will require a large investment of time, over a period of time, by the participants; and this in turn is going to require a more accommodating understanding by center management.

This issue leads directly to the broader question of the center's commitment to OD and to institutionalizing OD at MLK. This does not, to restate, mean setting up a formal department. It does suggest the need for a formal policy on OD that is understood throughout the organization, backed by both a long and short range plan for implementation, as well as a real sense of organization ownership. Specifically with reference to training OD resources, the center needs to have a policy with respect to (1) the utilization of internal OD resources (who, for what, how often, how much time, etc.), and (2) the training of present and future groups of OD resources (how many, how often, at whose initiative, by whom, etc.).

Implicit in these requirements are questions around the funding of trainers, the provision of release time, greater involvement in and understanding of the goals of OD training and of OD in general at the center, and greater involvement in seeing that those goals are met. Further, a commitment to developing an OD capability implies a commitment to utilizing OD technology in the conduct of the center's everyday activities. If OD is to work at lower levels in the organization, it is necessary that the higher levels be seen as living by the same rules. Thus, team development activities for top management should reflect commitment to OD. And greater involvement of lower levels of the organization in decisions affecting them would be particularly important.

To close with an example, it may be appropriate for the next group of OD trainees to have some input into the decision making process by which they are selected for this training, as opposed to the arbitrary selection process we experienced in this first round. The rationale here is that more self-selection is likely to result in participants who have a greater interest in and more commitment to OD. This, we suspect, would increase the chances of the trainees developing into competent OD resources.

# Appendix B

*TO:* *MLK Top Management*
*FROM:* *Irv Rubin and Mark Plovnick*
*SUBJECT:* *Basic Work Team Intervention* *Date: June 21, 1972*

The concept of the basic work team (BWT) structure evolved out of the center's continuing efforts to upgrade the quality of comprehensive health care delivered to the community. In order to better understand the potential usefulness and problems of the BWT structure (one family health worker and the part-time services of a public health nurse, a pediatrician, and an internist), and to facilitate its introduction to the center, MLK utilized its own internal resources in organization development. Each experimental BWT was assigned two or three trainee consultants to help implement the new team structure and to gather their own and BWT members' impressions about the viability of the concept as it actually operated on the teams. This report represents a summary of those impressions.

**Initial Contract: Objectives**

In some teams the BWT structure existed informally prior to the OD interventions. The experimental goal of the intervention was to formalize the structure with four BWTs. Specifically this goal included

1. To help the BWTs recognize themselves as a unit within the larger existing health teams.
2. To help them decide what they need to "team" about–i.e., for what purpose do they need to meet together as a four-person BWT.
3. To help them define appropriate roles for each of the four members–i.e., specifying members' operational responsibilities and limitations.

An outcome of these objectives would be a better understanding of the problems and benefits of the BWT structure. Further, in the process of functioning as facilitators in this intervention, the center's OD resources would gain considerable experience in their new role.

To accomplish these objectives the consultant teams contracted with their BWTs to engage in an action-research program of data collection, data feedback, and action planning. Specifically this included

1. A half-hour interview with each BWT member to gather his/her views on the organization, problems and potential of the BWT.
2. At least three sessions, 2–3 hours each, in which the BWT members and consultants engaged in (a) data feedback and diagnosis, and (b) action planning around the issues identified.

### Diagnosis of the BWT

Trainee consultants were asked to look at the BWT's goals, roles, processes, and interpersonal relationships, concentrating on the first two areas. Problems identified in the work with the BWTs, and in the center's health teams in general, can be understood within this framework. We will now look briefly at these four issues.

**Goals:** A team's goals should be clear to all members and shared by them. In the center, virtually everyone shares the goal of improved health care delivery to the community. However, in many cases this goal has taken on an inconsistent operational definition. In particular, the conflict between the quantity and the quality of care delivered is widespread in the teams. In large part this conflict seems to reflect ambivalence in the center's management with respect to the goal of quality care and the resource constraints the center faces. The ambivalence is translated to the teams in terms of "mixed messages," which specify not goals and constraints but procedures for meeting both. Because of the seeming inconsistency in these procedures, teams are often unclear about their priorities and thus spend a great deal of time and energy trying to understand, or guess, the underlying goals and constraints toward which they should be directing themselves.

A possible alternative for center management is to specify goals and resource constraints to the teams and, as far as possible, encourage teams to develop their own procedures to meet the stated objectives. For example, the center could specify an objective of a 10 percent increase in the number of patients seen per month while maintaining the quality of care, and let the individual teams find their own methods for accomplishing this. The benefits of this approach would be (a) a clearer understanding of the specific objectives, (b) procedures or solutions more appropriate to the particular set of circumstances facing each team, and (c) greater ownership of and commitment to the procedures developed by the team.

**Roles:** One of the most consistent observations made on the BWTs concerned the public health nurses' anxiety over their frequently changing and currently ambiguous role in the center. The conflict and ambiguity associated with the nurses' role results in anxiety for other team members as well. This general level of tension is in itself dysfunctional and debilitating, and often results in unnecessary conflict and resistance to changing procedures.

Part of the problem associated with the nurse's role can be traced to the manner in which the role changes were introduced. For example, instead of eliminating her supervisory responsibility for the family health worker by edict, each team might have been asked to work out a more equitable distribution of responsibilities, which at present were overburdening the nurses on some teams. This could have resulted in adopting different role strategies where appropriate; and in all cases, nurses and family health workers would have a better understanding of both the need for a role change (if any) and the nature of the new roles that developed.

Another issue centers around the feasibility or realism of the "ideal" family health worker role. The notion of the family health worker "managing" a family's health care met resistance from many MDs, nurses, and family health workers themselves. Doubts were raised about the FHW's skills as well as her desire and/or capacity to exercise the leadership necessary to fill the role of health manager. This suggests the need for a reorientation around the family health worker role, and/or new training for her. For example, training techniques are available for increasing self-confidence and assertiveness. Training in organizing and conducting meetings and conferences would also be useful in enabling the family health worker to assume some of the responsibilities involved in "managing" the team's resources in the delivery of family health care.

The natural dominance of the MD role was, and is, apparent to all those directly involved with the teams. One way to take advantage of this "given" is to use the physicians' leadership potential in teaching other team members skills that could result in greater total team participation and effectiveness.

Finally (again with respect to the physician), it appears unrealistic to assume that in addition to the current work load, he can spend large amounts of time each day meeting in each of the BWTs with which he would be involved. This suggests the need to further specify issues around which the physician would need to work with the BWTs.

**Processes.** One repetitive theme coming out of the interventions centered around the need for more problem solving skills on the teams. All BWTs complained about the time crunch, i.e., "we never finish anything," or "we don't have enough time to do everything," or "we seem to run up against the same problems over and over again." Effective problem solving requires widely shared skills in leadership, observation, listening, and intervention, as well as some familiarity with problem solving models.

In learning the new skills described, particularly the intervention skills, individuals and teams will also need to learn to take risks and experiment more. The teams observed were characterized by risk aversion. This posture, which may be functional in dealing with some health problems, prevents teams from finding new ways to deal with the *management* of health care delivery. An overabundance of rules and procedures passed down from the center's top management to the teams acts as an impediment to experimental behavior by causing confusion between means and ends (procedures and goals). As recommended earlier, more involvement by the individual teams in developing procedures for meeting center objectives could alleviate this confusion and lead to more experimentation.

**Interpersonal Relationships.** Problems between people, which are often erroneously attributed to "personality" clashes, most of the time are explainable in terms of difficulties with roles and/or processes. Thus, tension over the nurse's role ambiguity can lead to clashes between nurses and family health workers that have little to do with personality problems. This is probably what is happening in the frequently encountered perception that certain team members are seen by their fellows as "incompetent," both technically and interpersonally, and as such cannot perform the required functions of the BWT role. In some cases this might be true in the narrowest sense, but we suspect that a redefinition of the roles and relationships on the particular BWT could go a long way toward overcoming this problem. In most cases, increased skills in group processes, as described earlier, could eliminate the source of many interpersonal issues.

For those problems that do represent personality clashes, increased skill in confronting conflict and negotiating interpersonal settlements would help team members to work together, if not to actually like each other. The chances are that once people find they can work together, they also find they can get along with each other.

### Evaluation and Recommendations

In all four cases the consultants were able to facilitate the formal recognition and organization by team members of the basic work team structure. The four experiments differed in the extent to which they were able to focus on and solve issues central to the BWT. The following general recommendations are based on the preceding diagnosis of team effectiveness and on our own analysis of the results of this experiment.

**The Experiment.** One difficulty is that the basic work teams were taken out of their total team context for the purpose of this experiment. Thus, our observations often overlook the larger system implications of the BWT concept. For example, while MDs had little difficulty meeting for several hours per week with one BWT, it would be very difficult to meet with each of the six BWTs they would be associated with for comparable amounts of time. Therefore, we would recommend an experiment in which an entire health team is structured along BWT lines (i.e., the team has six BWTs).

An experiment of this nature would enable us to identify problems and benefits associated with relationships among different BWTs on the same team and among the BWTs and the larger team. We would also be able to focus on the problems of multiple BWT membership by MDs and nurses and on the need to differentiate BWT and total team issues.

### Team Performance

The experimental basic work teams were able to address themselves to—and often to solve—issues around goals, roles, and processes. This suggests that further interventions into the teams can be useful. Specifically, issues of problem solving, leadership, and role negotiation should be worked on. Because of their demonstrated ability to facilitate in these areas, the internal OD resources could be used (as some have already contracted to do) to help the teams work on these issues and further develop skills in these areas. A specific recommendation would be to work separately with groups of MDs, nurses, or family health workers to develop awareness and competence in required areas, while continuing to work on integrating the skills of the team members on the BWT.

Earlier we recommended specific training for MDs and family health workers, which could be examples of the training we are describing here. Training in homogeneous groups has the advantage of being more lasting for the individual than team training because of the rapid turnover found on the teams. However, facilitators in team meetings would still serve the much needed function of helping team members to utilize newly acquired knowledge and skills in team interaction.

With respect to the problem of rapid turnover on the teams, there is a need for a mechanism to integrate new team members into the team structure more rapidly and effectively. Currently the new member's socialization process is one of "sink or swim," with little attention paid to facilitating the process. Several alternative ways of dealing with this problem are available. One is to develop indoctrination programs or guidelines for teams to draw on in bringing new members on board, and to legitimize this activity by providing "slack" time for teams with new members. Another alternative is to develop centerwide socialization programs for new members to attend prior to joining their teams.

**OD Resources**

To enable the internal OD resources at MLK to play an expanding role in team development and other activities in the center, we recommend continued training for the current group, at their initiative, when the need arises; we also recommend that a similar program in skill training be started for a new group of potential OD resources to expand the number of such people available at MLK. A fruitful source of OD recruits would be the internship and residency program in social medicine at Montefiore.

**General Center Management**

To facilitate changes in the organization's structure and to increase individual skills in the effort to continuously improve the level of health care provided by the center as well as to provide a fruitful testing ground for innovations with national relevance, an atmosphere conducive to experimentation and growth is needed. The center's management can facilitate the development of this climate through its support of and participation in activities aimed at increased effectiveness through experimentation. To assist in coping with the problems of team delivery of health care, for instance, an experimental team might be established which would spend half its time delivering health care and the other half diagnosing and planning new methods of solving team problems. Such a team might also retain a full-time facilitator with OD skills. Operating in this manner over a period of several weeks could be sufficient to develop innovations impossible to discover in the pressurized environment that the teams now face.

Members of the center's top management can also further a climate of experimentation by attempting to develop new ways of working together as a team themselves, which would include exploring alternative methods of handling their relationships with other management levels at the center.

We believe our summarization of these global issues and our recommendations are consistent with our view that the center has reached a point where it is necessary to enlarge its perspective on organization change. Previous change efforts at the center have been useful in effecting some changes and in providing a great deal of information on the organizational dynamics at MLK. Based on this, we believe that the center is now ready and able to invest the time and energy necessary to undertake some of the efforts suggested here.

## About Chapter Five

*The impact of the MLK experience with organization development (whatever the outcome at the center turns out to be) is already evident in a number of other projects and programs. Techniques similar to those developed at MLK are being used by the National Health Service Corps to build health teams. Also, for the last year, the internship and residency program in social medicine at Montefiore has been training physicians to use some of the organization development techniques discussed in this book. Who knows, too, what other persons or institutions may have been influenced by reading an MLK annual report or hearing someone speak about the MLK experience with teams?*

*Yet at best we have taken only the first steps in a long journey leading into uncharted territory. Given our limited knowledge and experience, the question seems to be what priorities should be assigned for the immediate future?*

*Two that appear particularly urgent are: (1) to develop organization specialists who have a capability in the health care field, and (2) to train administrators and directors of health services in change agent skills so that traditional models of care in both hospitals and ambulatory centers can become more responsive to the needs of their patients.*

*Another critical dimension—and one of MLK's unachieved goals—is to involve the client more directly in the health maintenance process. In the ideal state, we believe, the patient and his family will be in charge of managing their own health care. Professional health workers would then function as technical assistants, facilitators, and counselors—supporting rather than controlling the family's management of its own health needs.*

*In Chapter Five, two programs looking to the future of the team delivery of health care are described. In Section One, Drs. Boufford and Kindig provide an overview of the Institute for Health Team Development at Montefiore Hospital. The goal of this program is to determine the educational methods and learning environments best suited to train interdisciplinary health science students to provide family-centered primary care as members of a health team.*

*In Section Two of Chapter Five, Richard Beckhard and Irwin Rubin describe the work the MIT group is doing in this area, including the creation of teaching materials that can be self-administered by teams, thus obviating the need to draw on scarce and expensive outside resources.*

*As we push into the future with these and other such projects, we are aware that the state of the art is primitive; that what we don't know is vast indeed compared to what we can lay certain claim to. So we light our candles against the dark. Perhaps what they illumine will provide the basis for another slim volume on making health teams work.*

*—Harold Wise*

# Chapter Five

# Next Steps

Section One
*Jo Ivey Boufford and David Kindig*

Section Two
*Irwin Rubin and Richard Beckhard*

## SECTION ONE: INSTITUTE FOR HEALTH TEAM DEVELOPMENT—THE NEXT TWO YEARS

The Institute for Health Team Development, located in Montefiore Hospital and Medical Center in New York City, is involved in working out a curriculum for the training of health science students from various disciplines whose goal is to provide family-centered primary care as members of a health team. The institute's work for the next two years has been funded by a grant from the Robert Wood Johnson Foundation. David Kindig and Harold Wise are co-directors of the Institute. Jo Ivey Boufford is director of education, with major responsibility also going to Richard Beckhard, Larry Platt, and Sue Eichhorn.

It is the hope of the group that this paper will stimulate comments and criticisms from others involved in health team development, for we seek continuing communication both from those who share our dream and from those who question its viability. And if our efforts should help to mobilize even a small number of people who are considering the use of teams in providing primary care, this paper will have more than fulfilled its purpose.

## GOAL

The goal of the Institute for Health Team Development is to establish educational strategies and learning environments that will prepare health science students from various disciplines to render comprehensive primary health services as members of health teams.

This report is a summary of a project, funded by the Robert Wood Johnson Foundation, to develop a school for health teams. Further information may be obtained by writing to Harold Wise, M.D., co-director of the Institute for Health Team Development, 3329 Rochambeau Avenue, Bronx, New York,10467.

Within this overall goal we have identified the following four objectives, which we hope to achieve in the next two years.

1. Identify and evaluate past experiences with health team training.
2. Develop effective educational methods and curricula for health science students who wish to learn how to deliver primary health care services through a health care team.
3. Carry out student health team training, testing educational models in various practice settings.
4. Serve as a focal point for coordination and communication of ongoing work in health team development.

Since we plan to use an action-research model in our work, objectives 2 and 3 will often be carried out simultaneously—that is, results of our work with student health teams will be fed back into curricular development, which in turn will be used in further team training efforts.

However, to get a better handle on the initial phases of implementing our educational goal, we plan to work in three areas: (a) developing the content to be taught to teams, (b) determining the best methods to teach it, and (c) locating and training faculty who will serve as both teachers and role models.

After we have developed and field tested several curricular approaches for the primary care training of student health teams in several different kinds of learning environments, we plan to make such curricula available to health institutions, which in turn might wish either to integrate the new material into their traditional curricula or set up new models of health education. Use of such curricula on any large scale could, we believe, initiate a major educational change effort, with potential long range impact on the way in which the health professional and client manage illness and health in the future.

## CONTENT

Our commitment, as we have stated, is to train interdisciplinary health science students as members of a team whose goal is the delivery of comprehensive primary care to patients and their families. We define a team as a group of health workers who must work interdependently to accomplish a task. The team in fact exists whenever a patient or his family requires two or more health workers to collaborate on his problem.

While such situations continually arise today, more often than not the required collaboration is far from effective. The fact is that health professionals, with the exception of the most structured situations such as the surgical team in the operating room, find it very difficult to work together. We believe there are good reasons for this. One of the most important is that the training of doctors, nurses, social workers, family health workers, etc., is generally confined to contacts with members of the same professional group. These people have little opportunity to get to know professionals from other disciplines until "professional roles" have been pretty much internalized. Furthermore, these professionals have not been taught *how* to work collaboratively.

The result is that students of various disciplines enter into patient care experiences with preset expectations of each other's roles and capabilities. Such expectations tend to lock into a continued cycle of traditional interactions between professional and professional, and professional and patient. This not only weakens the educational potential but also, ultimately, the service capabilities of health professionals–at the expense, of course, of the patient.

To break down this isolated training and the resulting stereotyping of health professionals, we plan to introduce the students, preferably early in their educational experience, to each other as members of an interdisciplinary health team. The content of their course in team training will be derived from a fairly clearly defined body of knowledge already existing in the fields of social psychology, group dynamics, and organization development. As members of a student health care team, they will deal with such issues as role definition and role negotiation, leadership, power, decision making, goal setting, joint planning, problem solving, open communication, and various team maintenance tasks.

**Primary Care**

The "vehicles" for such team learning, we believe, can best be taken from problems which relate to primary care practice within the family setting. We see at least two important educational advantages to this approach. First, while primary care is most often used to deliver medical care in the "real world," it is taught poorly if at all in most health education institutions today; the focus in these institutions is on disease rather than on a person with a network of needs relating to his illness. Second, since the primary care provider must bring together various areas of concern in his evaluation of the patient, what better way to construct a truly comprehensive picture than by making use of the multiple viewpoints and resources offered by the interdisciplinary team?

Let's take a look at health maintenance, since that will be an important concern of the team and will also provide a way for us to see how various team members function in a specific situation. First the team must develop and then monitor a set of parameters, both physical and psychosocial, to assess the family's state of health. This should require inputs from all team members. If one of these health maintenance parameters comes up abnormal, the team will be involved in a process of problem solving and solution implementation with the family to deal with the abnormality.

For some of the more common problems, the team might develop protocols or "standard operating procedures" so that team members will know what must be done as soon as an abnormality is uncovered and the protocol instituted. In other instances, because of the complex nature of the abnormality (especially if a psychosocial crisis is involved), the team will probably need to gather the necessary data and then proceed with a full scale conference to work out a management plan for the family. When possible, family members should be involved in the planning.

An example of team functioning set in motion by the discovery of an abnormal health parameter—in this case anemia in a three-year-old child at his regular checkup with the nurse practitioner—can be seen in Figure 5–1. The nurse would immediately discuss the finding with the pediatrician. In all likelihood a lead level test will be ordered because of the high incidence of children eating paint chips in this community. If the lead level comes back abnormally high, the child is referred directly to the team pediatrician. A problem-focused history is taken, a neurological exam is performed, and lab tests are checked. Though the child is asymptomatic, repeated tests and X-rays ordered by the MD reveal abnormally high lead levels and some deposits of lead in the child's bones. He will need to be admitted to the hospital for a week to ten-day course of therapy to remove the lead. The team then meets and begins instituting their "care plan"—which may be newly developed or part of a predetermined protocol for dealing with lead poisoning in children.

Whichever is selected, three problem areas will have been defined, each requiring work from different team members. First is the medical problem: the child has been hospitalized for treatment. The team pediatrician will stay in consultation with the hospital physicians and determine that lead detoxification is adequately completed. When the child is discharged, he will be rechecked periodically for lead levels and any signs of physical abnormality. The nurse practitioner will take responsibility for seeing that all other family members are screened for lead levels and that any abnormalities are reported to the team pediatrician or internist.

The second problem area is that of environmental hazard—the presence of lead paint in the home. To deal with this, the family health worker visits the home and takes samples of paint chips from walls and pipes and checks cooking and serving utensils for the possibility of lead-containing ceramic finishes. These are sent to the health department; if paint is positive for lead, the family health worker helps the client arrange for the apartment to be rehabilitated prior to the child's return home.

A third problem is the family's psychosocial situation. A possibility exists that the child's eating paint chips is symptomatic of childhood depression. To check on this, the family health worker might ask the social worker to make a joint home visit to do an in-depth family assessment of the child's position within the family constellation. The family health worker, who knows the family and the community, can provide invaluable information to the professionally trained social worker who is skilled in assessing complex family dynamics. If abnormalities are found here the two may wish to bring the problem back to the team to get other members' inputs in helping develop a plan for short and/or

**Figure 5–1.** Cycle of Team Functioning in Case of Anemia in Three-Year-Old

1. *FHW/Social Worker, student:*
*Primary data gathering*
*in routine home visit notes:*
(a) state of apartment
(b) family structure

2. *Nurse Practitioner, student:*
*Routine history, physical*
*and lab test reveal*
(a) anemia

3. *Team:*
*Anemia protocol instituted*
lead level > 60 mcg% (n. < 40)
*Problem formulation:*
1. Plumbism
2. Environmental Hazard
3. R/O Childhood Depression

4. *MD/medical student:*
*Problem focused history,*
*neurological exam, and*
*repeat lab work*
(a) lead level confirmed
(b) hospital referral needed

5. *Med. Consultant/*
*Hospital MD/*
*medical student:*
*Child hospitalized*
*for detoxification*
(a) hematology consult as needed
(b) family counseled on medical reason for hospitalization

6. *Team:*
*Care plan instituted*

A. *Immediate Treatment*
1. Medical. MD/PHN (a) hospital detoxification (b) other family members tested for lead
2. Environmental. FHW/PHN visit home; paint chips and cookware samples taken and sent to health department
3. Family Social worker/FHW
(a) in depth family assessment
(b) evaluate child's position in family dynamics

B. *Long Range Treatment*
focuses on patient education
1. Medical MD/PHN (a) periodic retest for lead (b) education on sources of lead and symptoms to watch for
2. Social worker/PHN/FHW Environmental—if paint is positive for lead, environmental repair of apartment or new apartment
3. Family Team (a) institute team plan for family treatment, e.g., therapy, day care for children, etc. (b) family counseling as to need for care

C. *Parameters to follow*
1. Lead level, symptoms—med. student/M.D. or nurse practitioner
2. Environmental repair—FHW/social work student
3. Family situation—FHW/social worker/PHN in consult with team

D. *Evaluation of Success*
1. No more lead levels
2. Home in good condition
3. "Family health" good

if abnormal, restart cycle

long term family therapy, day care, or other supportive counseling. Thus, team members (in this case the physician, nurse, family health worker, and social worker) work together with the patient and family to institute a comprehensive approach to managing the family's health problems.

While team members' roles and responsibilities will vary depending on whether the particular problem is lead poisoning, diabetes, hypertension, or whatever, in all cases a collaborative effort is needed to treat the disease as well as the psychosocial ramifications affecting the patient and his family.

In terms of the institute's team training objective, any such exercise in developing a comprehensive family care plan provides a vehicle for team members to experience the dynamics of team functioning. Indeed, team training will not focus on medical content per se so much as on understanding the team's own interactions. In other words, the team will study itself.

For example, if the primary care problem is management of a young diabetic, how does the team negotiate who is to be the primary practitioner for this patient? Will it be the doctor, who sets the initial insulin dose? Or the nurse practitioner, who will follow the patient when he is stabilized? Or the nutritionist, who is doing intensive diet regulation with the patient and his family? Or will primary responsibility shift from one person to another at different points? And if this is the case, how are the shifts negotiated? And how is the comprehensive treatment plan arranged? Have all team members made the necessary inputs? Who makes the decision as to how roles are negotiated? And how does the team determine to what extent the patient should be involved in these negotiations?

It is our contention that combining such primary care problems with an understanding of team dynamics will permit both faculty and student teams to look at the problems of primary care from a conceptual framework quite different from that which is now found in traditional health education institutions. For instance, rather than identifying a disease at one point in time, studying its pathophysiology, and treating its acute episodes in a hospital, the primary practitioner sees a patient with a medical problem at a certain stage which, in the normal course of events, is likely to progress in a more or less reasonably well defined pattern.

For example, let's look more closely at the case of a young diabetic just beginning to use insulin. In the near future he can expect a remission, with a resulting reduction in his insulin dosage. But after some period of normal life it is almost certain that he will return to insulin dependence. Although physically vigorous at the onset, in the 20 to 30 years ahead he faces the possibility of diabetic retinopathy, kidney disease, and cardiovascular complications resulting from his illness. What will the medical condition of the patient be at different points on such a continuum? How will his physical condition affect his psychological outlook? How will his psychological outlook affect his physical condition? What impact will all these realities have on his family, and on his own social and professional life? What kind of medical, personal, and social support systems will he need, and how can they be constructed before they are needed? Finally, what steps, if any, can his family take to prevent a replication or exacerbation of the medical and/or social pathology? How can team members help the family function as a more effective support system?

This kind of conceptual approach to health and disease is unique to primary care and is, in its richness, particularly well suited to collaborative team problem solving with the client and his family. Ideally, training in the use of this kind of approach should be initiated early in the student's experience and continue throughout his training. Furthermore, when team members have internalized an understanding of their own dynamics, and can effectively deal with team issues as they arise, more complex medical problems can and should be presented to the group.

**Family**

We have already stressed our concern for viewing the patient within the context of his family. By family we mean the support system for the patient, which might be his biological family and/or important others in his life.

The medical importance of the family has long been known, based on such work as genetic predisposition (sickle cell disease or diabetes mellitus); the transmission of infectious disease among persons living in close proximity (TB); and the apparent familial patterns of diseases such as hypertension and depression. There is also a growing body of knowledge indicating a social pattern of illness among family members, e.g., men with ulcers married to women with rheumatoid arthritis. And it seems likely this kind of sophisticated data will become increasingly available.

Recognizing the importance of the family, many primary care workers find that their major role lies in helping the family to cope with the patient's illness—in other words, maximizing the effectiveness of the patient's major support system, the family. To prepare for this, the health science student needs curricular experience in family studies relevant to primary care; he needs skills in assessing patient-family problems and in helping the family to manage its problems in illness and health; he needs a conceptual framework that will allow him to see every presenting patient within the context of his family. Such data will make it possible for him to determine the family's influence on the patient's illness and to identify possible resources within the family that can be mobilized to increase the potential for health.

To help team members develop such capabilities, we plan to prepare a series of team exercises that focus on family dynamics, beginning with the students own families. Our hypothesis is that given an understanding of their own dynamics, the students will develop the requisite skills to better understand the family dynamics of their patients.

For example, the team might be presented with the problem of a child who is "acting out" in school. To understand what is happening, the team members might participate in group exercises the goal of which is to analyze the family situation that led to the child's acting out behavior. This might involve the technique of "family sculpting" where team members play the roles of family members to try to understand the internal dynamics operating in the situation.

Making use of such knowledge, the team could then evolve a therapeutic plan for the family. The group could also use this opportunity to apply its training in team functioning to examine how this therapeutic plan has been negotiated. The team thus learns some basic concepts about families while still focusing on the team members' interactions in the problem solving process.

Again, as further research is done, larger pieces of content in family dynamics as well as methods of using family members as therapeutic resources can be developed and integrated into health science education.

## METHODS

We are committed to the experiential approach in terms of learning team dynamics. We think the data clearly show at this point that reading books about, or listening to lectures on, group dynamics are considerably less effective methodologies than experiencing a whole range of behaviors that exist in any group's interactions. Therefore, we focus on group "exercises," with team members examining their own interactions within the group.

In developing our curricula, we will depend on continued evaluation, feedback, and change whenever it is indicated. While team learning is our primary concern, at the outset we plan to obtain a personal "profile" of each team member, and, using various instruments, determine his or her most effective learning style. Such data, we believe, will be useful after team training to determine which types of individuals respond most favorably to the team experience.

Another major factor in educational methods is the learning environment. While it may be useful to look at the educational effectiveness of classroom vs. field experience, a more important methodological consideration, we believe, is to evaluate the *kind* of field experience or practice setting in which students will serve their educational apprenticeships. We hope to examine several different service models–hospital-based, health center-based, group practice-based, and private practice-based. Other variables will be urban vs. rural settings, as well as the appropriate mix of service vs. teaching time available to students and faculty in different settings. All these factors must be examined for their impact on the educational experience and the impact of the educational experience on the reality of service demands.

Another methodological consideration is the time frame for the team training experience. We plan to test several models. One that might be easily integrated into traditional health school curricula would be a relatively short experience (say three months) in team dynamics taken as an elective. More promising, we feel, would be continuing exposure to "teaming," which could make use of the increasingly complex medical material that students are being exposed to. This would permit integrating the student's clinical learning into the framework of primary care practice, which hopefully would make a positive contribution both to the student's service behavior and to his approach to other professionals.

Various combinations between brief limited exposure and continuous exposure to teaming will be tested. We will also be working with students at different stages in their training—first year students, those just beginning their clinical training, and perhaps some who have already completed professional school—to assess the effectiveness of the team experience at these various points.

Perhaps most critical of all in our educational strategy is the faculty. In no other field, we believe, is faculty so crucial as in the field of health sciences. Not only must such individuals be able to convey scientific medical knowledge, but in their interactions with patients and other health professionals they provide the role models on which the student will base his ideas of what is expected of him.

In our model, we plan to generate criteria for faculty selection early. We already know that the people we will be looking for will need to have experience as primary health care practitioners in medicine, nursing, or social service, as well as commitment to and skills in team functioning. We will also look for a strong interest in teaching.

But even with the best of backgrounds and deep commitment to our basic concept of family-centered primary care provided by an interdisciplinary team, we know that faculty training will also be needed. In fact, developing such a curriculum for faculty is a top priority in our work. And while the curricula developed will be similar for faculty and student teams, we recognize that with faculty we will have the added complexity of dealing with professionals who have already developed role habits.

These problems will be somewhat simplified by what we have learned from the team interventions at the Dr. Martin Luther King, Jr. Health Center and their evaluation by the MIT group. Also of help will be the materials for team training now being developed by Irv Rubin. And as our first faculty goes through team training, hopefully a methodology will evolve to train groups of interested faculty in more traditional institutions as primary care teams. These teams will then be able to train student health teams to deliver comprehensive care to patients and their families.

During this period we will also be examining the most effective mix of service vs. teaching time within the context of the educational and service demands on both faculty and students. The professional mix of faculty is another variable that may affect the model.

## OTHER ACTIVITIES

In addition to our major efforts in developing educational strategies for training interdisciplinary student health teams, the institute hopes to serve as a focal point for the coordination and communication of ongoing work in the health team area. Since the field is so new, we believe much of the existing information rests in pilot projects as well as the successes and failures of isolated individuals who do not know that anyone else shares their dreams. The Institute for Health Team Development will attempt to locate these people and bring them together periodically to share information and to assist in developing new hypotheses for the project. In addition, a newsletter or journal, containing current work in progress, book reviews, and letters, will be widely circulated. We will also be working in the field to increase knowledge and acceptance of the health team concept, particularly among those in key positions in hospitals and health care service institutions.

As the field develops, individuals who are skilled in the health team development process will be of critical importance for local consultation. Accordingly, we plan to hold workshops at least once a year for the training of trainers who can then impart health team educational methodology to interested professionals and students.

In the first part of the project, the major emphasis will be on program planning and development (see Fig. 5–2). The second phase—July 1974 to June 1975—will be primarily devoted to the major parts of field testing and training, with constant evaluation of content and methodology.

## EVALUATION

Evaluation of the most effective team training methodologies and experiences will be the critical element of the work. Only with careful and relevant evaluation will we be able to determine what future course to recommend to others—and to pursue ourselves—as more students are trained. The evaluation process will focus on the effectiveness of the various methodologies in imparting knowledge and facilitating attitudinal and behavioral change. The contents and processes of interdisciplinary teamwork will be evaluated in terms of their relevance to family oriented primary care. Since we will be working with students, and since the methodology is complex, no attempt will be made in this project to evaluate changes in the quantity or quality of the primary care given following interdisciplinary training.

Pre- and posttraining evaluative measures will be made of all trainees at all sites, including both objective and subjective assessments of content and process learning. Changes in each individual as well as the team as a whole will be critically examined in light of the particular training experiences. Although specific measures have not been selected, it is anticipated that they will include

**Figure 5–2.** Curriculum Development—Time Line for Project Activities

| *March 1973* | *July 1973* | *January 1974* | *July 1974* | *July 1975* |
|---|---|---|---|---|
| **1. Review and compile literature in the field of team.** | → | **1. Train first faculty team.** | ← | **1. Major field testing evaluation, modification and production of packaged materials.** |
| | | **2. Train first student team.** | | |
| **2. Investigate ongoing team training projects.** | → | | | |
| | | **3. Train 2–4 additional student/faculty teams with evaluation.** | | |
| **3. Determine faculty, student, and site selection criteria.** | → | | | |
| **4. Develop evaluation strategy.** | → | | | |
| **5. Develop first faculty and student curricular models.** | → | | | |

ome standard psychological and attitudinal tests, newly developed testing in interdisciplinary content learning, individual and team interviews, and observaion of team problem solving. As much early learning as possible will be fed into later training experiences in our action-research model.

The projected outcomes of our training effort will be several packaged curricular models for faculty and student education in team methodology, using the vehicle of family-centered primary care. In addition, we should have criteria for faculty, student, and site selection to help ensure the successful raining of student health teams. Finally, we hope to have organized a viable and convincing communications network connecting individuals and groups committed to the expansion of knowledge and expertise in the areas of team development and maintenance around the issues of primary care and family studies.

## SECTION TWO: EDUCATIONAL PROGRAMS FOR HEALTH MANAGEMENT

The growing need for better utilization of a variety of health workers in the delivery of comprehensive care is a significant aspect of the national concern about health care delivery. One model for more effective utilization of health manpower is the interdisciplinary team approach. Such teams, composed of physicians, nurses, social workers, family health workers, and lawyers, are emerging all over the country—in outpatient departments, community health centers, and group practice clinics.

The health workers' need for assistance in creating a more effective worker-patient relationship is a related issue for increasing numbers of physicians medical and nursing students, and health educators. Here the concern is to develop a global, patient oriented approach in the delivery of health care.

The need for the training and education of health workers in the facilitation and management of change is a third area of growing concern to increasing numbers of directors of community health centers, directors of health services, and program directors of community medicine. Organization development and other planned change efforts are currently being implemented in many health centers. Managers of such centers, as well as directors of teaching hospital and health schools and specialists in educational institutions, are seeking educational models and designs to help them in the management of change efforts.

In response to these needs, a three-part project has been mounted under the direction of Professors Beckhard and Rubin at the MIT Sloan School of Management. The creation of specific aids in the form of materials, curriculum plans, and development programs for use by administrators and program planner in the various health settings mentioned above are the goal of this project.

### Applying Knowledge and Experience from Other Settings to the Health Field

The behavioral and management sciences provide a body of knowledge which has been applied to individual and organizational effectiveness in other fields and is, we believe, particularly relevant to the health field. Specific areas applicable to the maximal development of skills and competence of health workers and managers are as follows.

This overview (based on MIT Working Paper #617-72, and prepared in the summer of 1972 describes a two-year program, funded by the Robert Wood Johnson Foundation, for the development of educational models for health workers and managers of health delivery institutions. Requests for further information should be directed to either Professors Richard Beckhard or Irwin Rubin, MIT Sloan School of Management, 50 Memorial Drive, Cambridge, Mass. 02139.

1. Knowledge and education in effective helping relationships.
2. Development of interpersonal competence and group membership skills.
3. Conflict management.
4. Decision making and problem solving.
5. Types and effects of different managerial styles and management strategies.
6. Diagnosis of client systems.
7. Organization development.
8. Facilitation and management of change.

The potential usefulness of these educational methods for health care institutions is borne out by the following: results obtained in improved organization and team effectiveness in a number of nonhealth settings; preliminary reactions from a variety of health professionals such as the American Association of Medical Colleges; and the positive effects of our intervention in some health delivery institutions. Specifically, in one urban health center the effectiveness of the delivery system as a whole, as well as that of the primary care teams, was improved by a series of educational interventions with interdisciplinary health teams, middle management, and top management.

Hard data on the number of patients treated, efficiency and accuracy of records, etc., are impressive. Measures such as the turnover of personnel, the proportion of time spent on care delivery vs. housekeeping and team maintenance have changed significantly. A number of jobs have been "enriched" and people have moved up in the organization more rapidly, increasing personal feelings of satisfaction at the health center. For example, one small group of center employees has been trained to act as internal change agents in facilitating future interventions. While quality of care has been maintained or improved, quantity of care has significantly increased, without additions to staff.

Our experience in this and other settings indicates that it is necessary to mount and manage a planned change effort if these results are to be achieved. Organization leaders and health workers who are members of such groups need specific educational help to do this.

## THREE SUBPROJECTS: A BRIEF DESCRIPTION

### 1. Interdisciplinary Team Effectiveness Program

Neighborhood health centers, the National Health Service Corps, and other organizations are making increasing use of interdisciplinary teams of health workers to deliver comprehensive health care. Extensive research on the dynamics of small groups, our own experience with task groups in a variety of settings, as well as our experience with health teams verify that there are a number of potential barriers to effective team functioning. Confusion over role responsibilities, decision making based on educational and professional status vs. who has the best information, distorted information flow between team members, and a lack of clear and shared team goals are burdensome and dysfunctional to the team. Often a negative cycle of events becomes operative: records are misplaced, patients are "lost," apathy grows. All of these impair the team's effectiveness.[1]

The prevalence of problems of this kind has made critics of the team approach conclude that, as they suspected, teams cannot work effectively. But the fact is that we know that teams in *any* setting are confronted with a series of issues and problems which, *if not effectively managed,* will operate to reduce their effectiveness. To assume that "nothing can be done about it" runs counter to a large and growing body of research and experience on the effectiveness of team development activities in a variety of settings including health care.[2] Rather than concluding that health teams don't work, the mistake has been to assume that "simply by calling a group a team, they will in fact behave like a team." The evidence is strong that before they can behave like a team, they need team training.

In this program, Professor Irwin Rubin and his colleagues will produce a set of guidelines for administrators and development specialists on strategies for introducing team development to health delivery and educational institutions. A series of learning modules or units will be developed to deal with identified aspects of team effectiveness for subsequent self-administration by health teams. Improved internal team functioning can release energy for a more direct and effective interface with patients. Thc modules will be field tested in two or three settings to assess their application under different circumstances, with their effectiveness measured against team effectiveness criteria.

### 2. Development of Internal Change Agents and Managers

The need for education and training in managing change has been demonstrated by health institution administrators, who are attempting to deal with the increasingly complex problems connected with today's environment. Physicians and other professional health workers who have moved into management positions in health care delivery institutions are recognizing that their preparation for the post has consisted mostly of technical training with virtually no management training.

Calls for more education of teams of health workers are increasing. The Student American Medical Association report "American Medical Education-the Student Viewpoint" makes the following "major recommendations":

1. Health care delivery should employ a multidisciplinary team of health professionals working to maintain health and prevent disease in communities, and members of these teams should be trained together in health universities.
2. Decision making should be decentralized to include administration, students, and consumers. The management of educational

institutions, curriculum administration, etc., requires skills in managing change, dealing with conflict, and problem solving.

Attention is now being focused on a reexamination of medical school curricula, with some movement toward selecting differentiated tracks for medical students after a core curriculum. Health care institution administrators, directors, personnel specialists, delivery team leaders, all feel an increasing need to understand the processes involved in managing change.

The purpose of this subproject, under the leadership of Professor Richard Beckhard, is to develop three specific curriculum programs:

1. Development of a program to train internal change agents, consultants, and organizational development specialists within a community health center from among health center staff.
2. An adjunct program for use by a house staff in a teaching hospital.
3. An educational program for use in medical, nursing, or other health schools.

To design these three curricula or programs we will recruit a "class" of professional health workers to field test preliminary material and to participate in the development of the final program. This "class," composed of physicians, nurses, dentists, social workers, and possibly other related health workers, will participate in a seminar or "course," using materials and formats which have been pretested for use in delivery and educational settings. Later, working within the interdisciplinary team structure, the participants will work on change projects in community health centers, outpatient departments, a National Health Service Corps team, a group practice setting, and a teaching hospital. This will enable participants and staff to evaluate those elements of their formal learning experience which they were able to use in their change efforts in the field. From this analysis will flow a better understanding of the course content and method necessary to train future change agents and managers in the delivery and educational settings specified above. Development of three separate curricula will proceed for field testing in some health schools, community health centers, hospital settings, and perhaps a group practice setting.

### 3. Health Worker-Patient Relationship

The training of most health care professionals (e.g., doctors and nurses) has emphasized clinical or treatment oriented skills. In other words, the focus has been on developing the requisite clinical knowledge to diagnose a disease and the technical skill to treat the disease once diagnosed. This knowledge and skill is, and will clearly continue to be, central to the delivery of health care.

However, the emergent focus of concern within the medical profession is on the patient and his total health care, as compared to the treatment of a particular disease. It has long been recognized within the medical profession that the more qualitative "human relationship" between health worker and patient is a significant component in the effective delivery of care. The importance of "bedside manner" (here meant to indicate a patient oriented rather than a disease oriented approach) is obviously not new. What is new is the acceptance of the idea that the development of certain qualitative human skills can be systematically taught rather than left to chance, or to personal identification with role models—e.g., senior physicians in a teaching hospital.

Our own experience in other settings clearly demonstrates that interpersonal skills and attitudes can be systematically developed.[3] Recent work by Abercrombie,[4] Lerner,[5] and others confirms both the relevance of these issues to the delivery of health care and the premise that they can be developed in "classroom" settings.

The interaction between a health worker and a patient, which should be an example of a helping relationship, often falls considerably short of the mark. Yet the acquisition of interpersonal skills and attitudes to make this relationship an effective one has been documented in a variety of settings. Health workers need knowledge and skills from several areas of the behavioral sciences—such as effective interpersonal communication, active/empathic listening, and dealing with the personal anxiety of the health worker—in order to develop a more patient oriented posture in their relationships with patients.

Program development in these areas by Professor Rubin and his colleagues is underway. Initial "experimental classes" will be composed of health workers directly concerned with the care of patients—i.e., doctors, nurses, nurse's aides, etc. These people will be drawn from a community health center and a hospital staff.

The final materials, designed for self-administration, are planned for use in on-the-job training situations, and will also be tested for relevance and integration into the ongoing curricula of health schools.

## THE TRANSFER OF KNOWLEDGE

Each of the subprojects described above represents an experiment directed toward meeting a specific set of health care related needs. In addition to the experiments with content, we will also be participant-observers in an experiment in the *process* of transferring knowledge from one field to another.

Our own project team, a core group of graduate students and staff from the Sloan School of Management, will work closely with an interdisciplinary support group tied into the project. The latter group includes the dean of a medical college, the director of a residency program in social medicine, a resident physician, and others. The advice, help, and support of many other yet-to-be-identified resources will also be important to the progress of these efforts. Experimental test sites for our team development and health worker-patient relationship educational modules will be particularly important. Participants in the program on managing planned change will have to be recruited from practicing health workers. Field projects will be located in delivery and educational institutions and project teams will be working together on real life organization improvement problems.

It is planned that in each of the three specific programs in the project, further utilization of the materials will be initiated in a variety of health settings. It is also planned that methods will be developed for testing the utilization of all three sets of products in all three settings.

## NOTES

1. R. Fry and B. Lech, "An Organizational Development Approach to Improving the Effectiveness of Neighborhood Health Care Teams: A Pilot Program." Sloan School, Masters Thesis, 1971; I. Rubin and R. Beckhard, "Factors Influencing the Effectiveness of Health Teams," Sloan School Working Paper No. 543–71, 1971. See also Chapter Two of this volume, which is based on material from the Fry and Lech thesis.
2. Fry and Lech, *op. cit.*; Rubin and Beckhard, *op. cit.*; *Fifth Annual Report: Martin Luther King, Jr. Health Center,* Bronx, New York; A.W. Parker, "The Team Approach to Primary Health Care," Monograph No. 3, Neighborhood Health Center Seminar Program, University of California at Berkeley, January 1972.
3. D. Kolb, I. Rubin, and J. McIntyre, *Organizational Psychology: An Experiential Approach,* Englewood Cliffs, N.J.: Prentice-Hall, 1971.
4. M.L.J. Abercrombie, *The Anatomy of Judgement,* London: Penguin Books, 1970.
5. M.J. Lerner, "Teaching Medical Behavioral Science: A Social Psychological Introduction," *Social Change: Ideas and Applications,* Vol. 1, No. 4, 1971.

# Contributors

Richard Beckhard
Jo Ivey Boufford, M.D.
Ronald E. Fry
David Kindig, M.D.
Aileen L. Kyte
Bernard A. Lech
Thomas F. Plaut, M.D.
Mark Plovnick
Irwin Rubin, Ph.D.
George A. Silver, M.D.
Harold Wise, M.D.

# Bibliography


Argyris, Chris, *Intervention Theory and Models,* Reading, Mass.: Addison-Wesley, 1970.

Beckhard, Richard, *Organization Development; Strategies and Models,* Reading, Mass.: Addison-Wesley, 1969.

Bennis, W., Benne, K., and Chin, R., *The Planning of Change,* New York: Holt, Rinehart and Winston (2nd ed.), 1969.

Harrison, R., "Role Negotiation: A Tough Minded Approach to Team Development," Development Research Associates, unpublished.

Horowitz, John J., *Team Practice and the Specialist,* Springfield, Ill.: Charles C Thomas, 1970.

Kolb, David and Frohman, Allen, "An Organization Development Approach to Consulting," *Sloan Management Review,* Cambridge, Mass.: MIT, 1970.

Kolb, David; Rubin, Irwin; and McIntyre, James, *Organizational Psychology: An Experiential Approach,* Englewood Cliffs, N.J.: Prentice-Hall, 1971.

Lawrence, Paul and Lorsch, J., *Developing Organizations: Diagnosis and Action,* Reading, Mass.: Addison-Wesley, 1969.

McCormack, R. and Wise, H., "A Pilot Training Program for Primary Care Practitioners of a Health Team," 1970 (unpublished).

MLK Health Center, "Your Rights As a Patient," A general community curricula, 1970.

Miles, Matthew B., *Learning to Work in Groups,* New York: Teacher's College Press, 1959.

Moynihan, D.P., *Beyond the Melting Pot,* Cambridge, Mass.: MIT Press, 1964.

Parker, Alberta W., *The Team Approach to Primary Health Care,* Berkeley, California, Neighborhood Health Center Seminar Program, 1972.

Revans, R.W., *Standards for Morale: Cause and Effect in Hospitals,* London: Oxford University Press, 1964.

Rubin, Irwin and Beckhard, Richard, "Team Effectiveness Model and Immediate Next Steps: A Working Proposal," 1969 (unpublished).

Schein, E.H., *Organizational Psychology,* Englewood Cliffs, N.J.: Prentice-Hall, 1965.

Schein, E.H., *Process Consultation,* Reading, Mass.: Addison-Wesley, 1969.

Silver, George A., *Family Medical Care,* Cambridge, Mass.: Harvard University Press, 1963.

Walton, R.E., *Interpersonal Peacemaking: Confrontations and Third-Party Consultation,* Reading, Mass.: Addison-Wesley, 1969.

Wise, H., "Third and Fourth Annual Report: Dr. Martin Luther King, Jr. Community Health Center," 1969, 1970, New York: MLK Health Center.

# Index

# About the Authors

**Harold M. Wise** is Director of the Internship and Residency Program in Social Medicine at the Montefiore Hospital. He is also co-director of the hospital's Institute for Health Team Development, as well as Associate Professor of Community Health at the Albert Einstein College of Medicine. He was founder and first director of the Dr. Martin Luther King, Jr., Health Center. He received his medical training at the University of Toronto. His early involvement in community medicine began in Canada with the development of a consumer cooperative health clinic using the health team approach.

**Richard Beckhard** is Senior Lecturer in Management at the Sloan School of Management at MIT and adjunct Professor of Social Psychology at Teachers College, Columbia University. He is also a consultant in organizational behavior and development for many American and international firms.

**Irwin M. Rubin** is Senior Lecturer in Organizational Psychology at the Sloan School of Management at MIT and a consultant to a number of companies, foreign governments, and departments of the American government. He received his Ph.D. in organizational studies from MIT.

**Aileen Kyte** is a free lance editor and writer specializing in the field of behavioral science and organization development. Prior to her assignment in the preparation of this book, she served as an editorial consultant at McKinsey & Company.